FIX YOUR
FATIGUE

The four-step process to resolving chronic
fatigue, achieving abundant energy and reclaiming
your life!

Evan H. Hirsch, MD, ABOIM
with Stacy Scheel Hirsch, MES, ACC, CDWF

Additional Resources

FREE bonus material in our membership site at FixYourFatigue.org/members

JOIN our Facebook community! Get answers to your questions at FB.com/groups/FixYourFatigue

If you want to become a patient at my clinic, please go to TheHirschCenter.com and begin the new patient process. We see patients from all over the world.

Feedback

P.S. If this book helped you, please let others know that there is a way out of fatigue and post a short review and your success story on Amazon at https://goo.gl/pFFe0y. I will be eternally grateful!

P.P.S. Your support makes a difference and I read and respond to every review personally so I can make this book even better.

P.P.P.S. If you DON'T like the book, send me an email and tell me why. I will thank you for the feedback and gladly refund your money. Okay? You can email me at feedback@fixyourfatigue.org.

P.P.P.P.S. If you find any spelling, grammatical or layout errors in this book, please email me at the above email address with the page number, sentence, and mistake, and I'll fix it right away and be so grateful for your help! I want to make sure this book is the best it can be for you and everyone suffering from fatigue.

If you're a provider and you want to be trained by me, please email me as well.

Get Connected!

Here are the links if you want to follow me on social media:

Facebook:
https://www.facebook.com/DrEvanHirsch/

Twitter:
https://twitter.com/drevanhirsch

YouTube:
https://www.youtube.com/c/evanhirschmd

LinkedIn:
https://www.linkedin.com/in/drevanhirsch

Google+:
https://plus.google.com/+EvanHirschMD

Testimonials

"Dr. Hirsch's program is a lifesaver." - JzB

"After doing what Evan recommended I am a changed man. I feel better than I have felt in 20 years. Feeling better has given me an optimism combined with energy like I haven't felt since I was in my 30's. I have been given a life like I never thought I would have again. Overall I feel 20 to 30 years younger (I'm 68). Thank you, Dr. Evan. I'll never be able to repay you for what you have given me." – M.S.

"My energy is better than it has been in years as is my capacity for physical exercise. My energy is up to a 7.5-8/10. I have also had a tremendous improvement in my memory as well." - L.S.

"If you want a solution to your complicated health problems and are willing to put in the effort you will see results like nowhere else. Take this rare opportunity to get the help you need. You will not be disappointed." - Pati

"Within a month of focusing attention on my true health issues - I've lost belly fat - I sleep much better - my energy level has improved - I'm coping with high stress levels without having to take conventional anti-anxiety medication - life just has a more positive spin - Thank You - for providing an alternative way to health!" - Janice

"Dr. Hirsch has helped me achieve much higher levels of energy, weight loss, pain reduction (from food allergies - dairy and gluten). I feel the clock has been reversed, as I now feel ten years younger than I did since I started seeing Dr. Hirsch three or four years ago. I have also had resolution of the depression, the fatigue, and the brain fog -- I am more focused, organized and alert. Thank you Dr. Hirsch for your help!" - T.S.

"After seeing Dr. Hirsch for four years, I can honestly say this is the best I have felt in a very long time. I do not have anxiety like I did, it is well maintained now. I have more energy, my moods are stable, and I feel like doing things and going places. Since I have been under Dr. Hirsch's care, I now have not needed my asthma medicine in over a year, and my allergies have gone to almost nothing. I was the type of person who took all kinds of medicine almost every day just to get by. I worry about my throat closing from my allergies, and I can honestly say I really don't even think about that anymore. I have to thank Dr. Hirsch from the bottom of my heart because I feel like I have a life again." - J.M.

Disclaimer

The book is for informational purposes only. Neither the publisher nor the author is engaged in rendering professional advice or services to the individual reader. The ideas, procedures, and suggestions contained in this book are not intended as a substitute for consulting with your physician. All matters regarding your health require medical supervision. Neither the author nor the publisher shall be liable or responsible for any loss or damage allegedly arising from any information or suggestion in this book.

While the author has made every effort to provide accurate telephone numbers, Internet addresses, and other contact information at the time of publication, neither the publisher nor the author assumes any responsibility for errors, or for changes that occur after publication. Further, the publisher does not have any control over and does not assume any responsibility for author or third-party websites or their content.

This book is dedicated to my wife, Stacy,
for teaching me about fatigue,

my daughter, Selah,
for being my motivation to prevent fatigue in others,

and to all those who suffer from fatigue.

Acknowledgements

This book would not have been possible without the amazing people I have in my life.

I'd like to start by thanking my wife and best friend, Stacy. Thank you for encouraging me to grow and for holding space for my process, the rewards have been great. Thank you for the beautiful chapter you wrote. It is going to help so many people. I have never met anyone who can accomplish more in a day, throw together amazing meals in an instant, support patients emotionally, teach our employees about their emotional health and love me as well as you do. I am so lucky you emailed me back. I love you. Thank you, my dearest friend.

To my daughter, Selah, the love I have for you is endless. I am so grateful for all of our moments together. May you always be blessed with a song in your heart, a story on your mind, a piece of paper for your art and a creative space for your dreams. Thank you for your patience while I wrote this book. We can now start reading Harry Potter together again.

To my parents, Sydney and Jerry, thank you for providing me a great upbringing, a college education, and your love.

To my siblings, Janine and Tovah, thank you for always being supportive of my dreams and for your hugs.

To Donna Mosher, my editor, thank you for being my cheerleader and for all of your advice and patience in making this book such a gift for those with fatigue.

To Valerie Burke, MSN, thank you for taking the dictations from my mouth and the research you found and converting them into words on a page. Without your help, this project would have taken a lot longer.

To Misha Kogan, MD, thank you for writing the foreword, my dear friend. I am always amazed at all that you create in your life and the way you hold space for spirit.

To my best friends Jared Adler, Mikey Madigan II, Alonzo Grant, Dave Nevy, Bobby Botnick and Ari Halpern thank you for all of your encouragement, support and love through the years.

To my office staff for always being so supportive of my vision and this project:

To Allison Hamza, PA-C, thank you for all of the ways you have supported me as a friend and colleague. Thank you for your words of encouragement and for taking care of our patients with such grace and compassion. Without knowing that our patients were well cared for in your hands, I truly could not have written this book.

To John Farinelli, thank you for all of your support in so many aspects of my life. Whether I needed you to manage a project, create a form or take a meeting for me, I knew you were going to be there and do it well. I am forever grateful.

To Pam Scheel, thank you for all you do at the office and for me personally to make my life better. I know I can always count on you.

To Kim Dahl, thank you for being my right-hand woman at the office, for managing my faxes, looking out for me, supporting our patients and making me look good.

To Angie Thompson, ARNP, thank you for all that you bring to our patients and our clinic, your curiosity, your compassion, and your search for the best tests and treatments available.

To Amanda Campbell, thank you for the smile and positive attitude you bring every day. The safe space you create for others is amazing.

To Lisa Bent, thank you for all of your hard work and dedication, your teasing and fun personality, and being open to new things.

To Gina Christensen, thank you for your positive attitude and for sending me home when I was procrastinating to finish this book.

To Virginia Hadley, thank you for all that you do for our patients, your compassion, your caution and your curiosity.

To Andrea Shamansky, thank you for staying up late to make sure I had the photographs I needed for the book cover. I am so grateful for your support!

To Jason Chafin, thank you for setting up and managing our online world and always doing so with a smile and a joke.

A huge debt of gratitude goes to all of my teachers, those known and unknown who have guided and supported my growth as a physician and human. Nothing that I discuss in this book is new; I have merely compiled the work of those who have come before me and made my own observations.

Finally, many thanks to all of my patients. You have taught me so much through our partnerships and healing breakthroughs.

I am truly grateful and blessed to share my life with such wonderful people.

Thank you all!

Table of Contents

Foreword

Dr. Evan Hirsch's new book on fatigue is concise, easy to understand, and a must-read for every person struggling with the debilitating symptoms of fatigue.

Evan and I met when we first embarked on our journey into the field of integrative medicine. We instantly became close friends, and since that time we have been exchanging protocols, learning from one another, and closely following each other's work.

Today, medical practices are challenged with patients suffering from chronic fatigue. Practitioners of integrative or functional medicine look beyond symptoms for the cause of a condition. Dr. Hirsch and I routinely see patients who have been ignored by conventional medical offices, especially when standard tests do not reveal any obvious abnormalities. These patients are frequently sent to psychiatrists or shuffled from one consultant to another, wasting valuable time and demoralizing people who are already suffering.

In *Fix Your Fatigue*, Dr. Hirsch guides you through the process he used to relieve his own fatigue. He shares the solutions he discovered that worked for him and that are working for the patients who are fortunate enough to work personally with him in his busy functional medicine practice.

Be forewarned; this is not a quick solution you may get from a pill. The journey is multi-faceted and extensive. But it is expedited by the trial and error Dr. Hirsch conducted himself to get results. It took years for him to identify what works. If you follow his guidance, you will save time and money.

The bonus? This book guides you not only to fix your fatigue, but in following his steps and recommendations, you will reclaim the overall health of your youth. This is everyone's birthright.

As a geriatrician, I'm well aware that chronic fatigue in the elderly not only causes suffering but shortens their lifespan and has high financial and emotional costs. It affects the individual and also those involved in their care. It doesn't need to be this way. Aging doesn't mean we lose our strength, energy, and vitality. There is a better way to age, and it doesn't involve fatigue.

The unique strength of Dr. Hirsch's book is that it is thorough while still presenting the information in an easy-to-comprehend format. Any patient at any age with fatigue who follows the steps outlined in this book will begin their journey back to health and back to reclaiming their life.

Mikhail Kogan, MD

Medical Director
George Washington Center for Integrative Medicine
www.integrativemedicinedc.com
Assistant Professor of Medicine,
Associate Director of Geriatric Fellowship

Introduction

One month into my family medicine residency training program, I met my wife, Stacy. She was full of life, socially active with many friends, a great cook, a traveler, a small-business owner, and committed to her personal growth through self-examination. Four months later, this active, vivacious woman was suffering from exhaustion. She had adrenal fatigue, and her cortisol levels (the primary adrenal hormone) were non-existent. A naturopathic physician diagnosed her with chronic fatigue. She was told to rest up, and she would be better in one to two years. Unfortunately, it took three years!

You can imagine how frustrated we felt. I was training to be a doctor, and I had no tools to help her. I felt powerless. Stacy purchased a sauna; she began taking adrenal supplements and coffee enemas, and she worked on her negative emotions and past trauma. Sure enough, she was *mostly* better in three years. But three years is a *long* time! I wanted to find a better and faster way to heal. So I began learning everything I could about fatigue.

After I completed my residency in 2007, I started my functional medicine practice. (Functional medicine addresses the underlying causes of disease, not just symptoms.) Stacy's fatigue symptoms were resolved. But now I realized that *my* energy wasn't like it was before residency. I was able to function, but I was tired. I didn't have much energy for exercise, nor did I prioritize it. I had worked long and hard for the opportunity to create my practice and to deliver the integrative health care I knew to be effective, so I pushed ahead. I assumed my fatigue was a post-residency issue that would resolve on its own in a few months.

Unfortunately, it didn't get better. With the birth of our daughter in 2008, my energy and brain fog started to worsen. I could see patients only part time; no more than six hours a day, four days a week. I had body pain. I couldn't remember much about my patients, and I had to rely on what was in their medical records. I was cold all the time. I lost my hair, and it became brittle and dry. I had no libido. My calves would cramp up for no reason, especially at night. My energy would crash at 3 p.m. every day. I would spend time with my daughter, but I wasn't able to access the joy I knew I should be experiencing. I wasn't much help at home, which made me feel guilty since my wife was shouldering the load. I couldn't manage my staff, and I couldn't afford to hire more to help. I increased my patient load to pay our expenses, but I knew it wasn't sustainable, so I hired other providers to allow me to decrease the number of patients that I was seeing. Every day it was a struggle just to get to work and provide excellent patient care. When I got home, I didn't have any energy left for my family. It wasn't a happy existence.

On a Search

As I went to conferences, studied books, and evaluated the research, I began to compile a list of causes of chronic fatigue. In medical school I was taught, "If you don't think of it, you won't diagnose it." I broadened my view to include all potential causes. A patient handed me an incredibly valuable resource; a copy of the book *Fatigued to Fantastic* by Jacob Teitelbaum, MD. Dr. Teitelbaum used the acronym S.H.I.N.E to illustrate the main causes of fatigue and fibromyalgia that he had found. S.H.I.N.E stands for Sleep, Hormones, Infections, Nutrient deficiencies, and lack of Exercise. I found this framework to be very helpful and expanded on it over the subsequent years with my own findings and research.

Many of these causes I was able to find in conventional medical textbooks, but conventional medicine lacked the testing methods to determine if they were causing the fatigue. In my functional medicine research, however, I could find the testing methods I needed to assess these potential causes. I implemented what I was learning in my practice and was very pleased with the success my patients experienced.

I trained with the Institute for Functional Medicine. Functional medicine, as I said, looks for the causes of disease and dysfunction and the areas of imbalance – not just symptoms. It looks at where our biochemical and physiologic processes have become abnormal and removes the problem or replaces the deficiency so the body can heal itself. It allows me to practice truly individualized medicine because no two people have same the causes of fatigue and they require different treatments to resolve their causes.

I found that there were still patients with fatigue that I couldn't help, so I kept searching for answers. I found many of my answers in the trainings offered by the American Academy of Environmental Medicine. It was there that I learned about the toxicities related to heavy metals, chemicals, molds, and electromagnetic frequencies.

The final piece of the puzzle (as I currently see it) was chronic infections. I read and learned from Richard Horowitz, MD, and his book, *Why Can't I Get Better? Solving the Mystery of Lyme and Chronic Disease.* The Institute for Functional Medicine had a conference that was helpful, and I trained with Nikolas Hedberg, DC, and his *Infection Connection* course.

As I implemented what I was learning, I saw amazing results. Many of my patients had suffered for ten years or more without success. As they got better, we cried together for the years they had lost to this debilitating illness. I vowed to help as many people suffering from chronic fatigue as I could.

My commitment to help others with fatigue expanded, and I realized my mission went beyond my clinic. I envisioned helping a hundred thousand people resolve their chronic fatigue! I never wanted anyone to suffer as my family, my patients, and I had.

As my patients got better, I finally began to treat myself as well. As I resolved my vitamin and hormone deficiencies, my energy increased from a 3 out of 10 (10 being ideal energy. See the Fatigue Scale at the end of the introduction) to a 6 out of 10. When I started treating heavy metals and chemicals, my energy improved to a 7 out of 10. Now, treating infections, molds, and improving my emotional health has raised my energy to an 8 out of 10.

After ten years of clinical practice, I have finally curated an effective, systematic approach to treating chronic fatigue that works. It is called the Fix Your Fatigue Program, and it has alleviated my fatigue and hundreds of my patients' fatigue so successfully that I am compelled to share it with you.

If you or someone you love is battling fatigue, you may have seen multiple healthcare providers without finding the cause and resolution to your symptoms. Maybe you've given up on ever feeling better, believing you'll just have to "live with it" for the rest of your life. If this is you, then congratulations—this book has the answers that will help you feel alive and vital once again!

This book is a compilation of my years of clinical experience, study, and personal experience with chronic fatigue. Please read it as a how-to manual. I have done my best to simplify the technical details and give you only the information that you need to be successful.

The Format of This Book

My goal is to give you the information you need to determine if you have a particular cause and how to treat it. Then you can act on these suggestions, get better and improve the quality of your life and the lives of those around you. This is my vision for your life.

I know you probably have brain fog and can't absorb and organize lots of material, so I have done my best to simplify, outline, and summarize the material while still giving you the information you need to understand the concepts. To that end, I created *Appendix B: Treatment Plans and Action Steps,* which contains all of *The Plan* and *Action Steps* from every chapter in the book for an easy reference. You can download this from the free membership site I have created for you (more on this in a little bit).

The chapters build on each other, so it is ideal for you to complete them in order. For example, you will be more successful at removing infections once you have started removing heavy metals, chemicals, molds, and emotions.

I recommend that you complete one chapter per week. This will give you the opportunity to focus on one issue at a time and see how you respond to treatment before addressing the next issue.

Did you know that when it comes to completing programs like this that 97 percent who purchase them never finish? This is because we lose our motivation and any complexity slows us down. This is why my goal has been to keep it simple and give you clear guidance.

I recommend that you focus on *The Plan* and *Action Steps* sections at the end of every chapter to help you be successful. If there are multiple Action Steps, I recommend that you start one every four to seven days so that you can see how your body responds to the treatments.

I start each chapter with a brief story of my experience or that of a patient I have seen (with the name changed, of course) that illustrates what we are going to discuss. I then go on to discuss the *Background*, *Symptoms*, *Testing*, and *Treatment* sections. At the end of each chapter, the *Summary*, *The Plan*, and *Action Steps* sections are probably the most helpful because they summarize the most important points and discuss the exact steps you need to take to implement treatment. If you have brain fog, focus on these sections to save time and energy.

These protocols have proven themselves time and time again to be effective. I have the utmost confidence that they will help you as well!

Additional Support for You

I have created a closed Facebook group (fb.com/groups/fixyourfatigue) to support each other through community. There is a lot of research on the benefits of community, and our Facebook group will offer that. Introduce yourself when you get there and share what you're going through. Ask and answer questions and always be supportive, patient, and compassionate. I think you'll find it to be a very rewarding experience.

I also created a free membership section of my website (fixyourfatigue.org/members) to hold the resources mentioned throughout the book. Take advantage of these free tools to get the most out of this book. I truly believe that the more you use these support tools, the more successful you will be.

Laboratory Tests

I encourage you to work with a medical practitioner, preferably one trained in functional medicine. You will be able to achieve results more quickly when you have a healthcare partner. I will be recommending laboratory tests to assist in assessing your causes of fatigue and monitoring treatment. A healthcare provider can facilitate the acquisition and interpretation of these labs and any nuances to your treatment that are beyond the scope of this book.

If you are not able to work directly with a health care provider, there are some resources that you can use. You can order many of the blood tests that I recommend from FYF.MyMedLab.com and some of the specialty (functional) labs from DirectLabs.com. I am not compensated for recommending these labs to you. You will need a provider for any labs that I recommend that are not found on these sites.

When evaluating laboratory tests, it's important to note that most local laboratory ranges are based on the total number of people who took the test and not on what is optimal. Consequently, I will include my recommended laboratory ranges for you to use. I generally will use the reference ranges given by the functional medicine laboratories.

I recommend that all blood labs be completed first thing in the morning (preferably before 9 a.m.) and that you fast for them. Drink lots of water for the twelve hours leading up to the blood draw, but no food after midnight. Consider bringing your breakfast to your blood draw so that you can eat after you are done.

Fatigue Scale

Through this book, you will find references to a fatigue scale, which you will use to assess your progress. I recommend that you use this scale with the Symptom Calendar that you can download from the member area (fixyourfatigue.org/members). Every day, mark on the calendar where you are on the scale. I use a scale from 1 out of 10 (1/10) to 10 out of 10 (10/10).

1/10 – Can't get out of bed

2/10 – Can get out of bed and walk around the house a little

3/10 – Can take care of the basic needs at home, but not enough energy to leave home. Can dress oneself, but needs to rest often

4/10 – Can take care of more advanced needs at home – cook meals, pay bills, etc., – but not enough energy to leave home

5/10 – Able to get out of the house, but not much else (can go to only one appointment a day)

6/10 – Able to get out of the house and has energy throughout the day with a few crashes

7/10 – Able to get out of the house with mostly sustained energy through the day, can exercise a little bit without feeling worse or crashing

8/10 – Sustained energy throughout the day and able to exercise moderately without crashing

9/10 – Sustained energy throughout the day and able to exercise intensely without crashing

10/10 – Sustained energy throughout the day and able to exercise intensely or lose sleep for periods of time without crashing

Expectations

So, this is a good time to talk about expectations.

1. First, this book is a guide only. I am not offering medical advice. This book is for educational purposes and based on my clinical and personal experience with fatigue. I highly recommend that you work with a health care provider knowledgeable in functional medicine to deal with all the nuances you will experience on your healing path.

2. Using my protocols does not mean we have a therapeutic relationship. I can only practice medicine in Washington State, and unless I've seen you in person in my practice, we do not have a doctor-patient relationship.

3. My protocols are not guaranteed to work. They have worked on hundreds of patients with fatigue, but sometimes they don't work. Most of what I am addressing in this book are those issues on the physical level (your body), and often individuals need support on the energetic, emotional, psychological, and spiritual levels. Stacy (my wife and author of the chapter on emotions) and I will be addressing these in the book, but sometimes the work on these levels requires more time. I highly recommend that you find support – a good therapist, energy healer, Reiki master, psychologist or health coach – to help resolve any of these issues, because it will be very hard for you to get better if you do not address these barriers.

4. I don't expect you to be perfect. I'm definitely not. I expect you to struggle with drinking enough water or staying away from sugar or remembering to take all of your supplements. It's hard, and you may blow it. I don't want you to beat yourself up over it. You are human. I want you to have compassion with yourself, forgive yourself and then re-commit to the process. I have provided you my Treatment Schedule and Calendar (in the member area) to help you keep track of your treatments and stay on course.

5. You won't get better just by taking supplements. You'll need to increase your exercise over time, change the food you eat, work on your psychological issues, create goals for yourself, and develop gratitude and a positive attitude.

6. Your progress is going to be up and down. You're going to have "bad" days when you don't feel well, after several "good" days. You're going to think that the treatment isn't working and that you should change or stop it. Don't do it! These changes are part of the process. We're looking for baby steps in the right direction. Sometimes this looks like two steps forward and one step back. Our goal is for *more good days* per week until eventually, all your days are good! The body is adjusting to these changes, and it can be uncomfortable. We are creating a new normal for the body, and it takes some getting used to.

7. Getting better takes time. The body likes small changes, and depending on the number and types of causes you have, complete resolution can take six months to two years. Stay the course and trust this process; you will get better.

8. You won't get better if you can't balance acceptance with perseverance. You need to accept where you are, have gratitude for your life and your situation, but not settle for it. You need to continue forward and remain committed to taking your supplements and maintaining good lifestyle practices.

9. You won't get better without the right tools. It has taken me ten years to find the right supplements at the best prices. Don't lose time and money by trying to find less expensive supplements. They usually don't work and end up costing you more (in time and money) in the end. It's incredibly unfortunate when a patient isn't getting better, and it's all because the supplements they are taking aren't working.

Please note: you definitely do not have to purchase your supplements from me, but I have setup an online supplement store for you with all of the products that I recommend in this book. In this store, you will get 5% off every order. You will also get free shipping when you spend more than $50.

Full Disclosure

I make money off the sale of this book, my supplement store and some of the products that I link to in this book. If you purchase these products through the links I provide, the cost to you remains the same as if you purchased it elsewhere, and I get a referral fee. Thank you for supporting me and my mission!

People who Shouldn't Read This Book:

This book is not for everyone. I only want people to read this book who are committed to resolving their fatigue.
You should **NOT** read this book if:

1. You're looking for an instant, easy fix. This process takes time and dedication.

2. You're not interested in changing your diet or bad habits.

3. You're not coachable. You don't want to make the changes that I'm recommending.

4. You need references and research to back up everything that I say. Almost everything I recommend has research behind it, but some of it doesn't. All of it is based on my clinical experience of what works. You can find the research in the Reference section at the end of the book.

5. You're not able (because of cost, etc.) or willing to take supplements. They are one of the main tools I use to help people heal.

6. You're not sure if you want to get better because then you might be asked to help out with other things or go back to work.

7. You're not committed to working on any emotional issues that may be present.

8. Your family represents a barrier to making changes in your life. For example, you're not able to change your diet if your family objects.

If the above list does not describe you, then this book is for you! Whether you're a patient with fatigue or a physician who wants to help patients recover from fatigue, this book is a roadmap for getting well. It is a tool to help you get back on your feet and to live your life with energy and passion. In this book, you will find a practical nuts-and-bolts guide to fixing your fatigue. Follow my years of training and personal experience, and you will be successful.

Resolving your fatigue and restoring your energy requires a commitment. You, your family, and your kids are worth it! After you complete the program and you have all the energy you need to enjoy your life, you will look back on these days of exhaustion with amazement that you could ever feel so tired. You will be filled with gratitude that your body can deliver such vitality. Fixing your fatigue *will change your life*.

Ready? Let's get started!

Chapter 1:
The Causes of Chronic Fatigue

As a physician, I have found chronic fatigue to be one of the most common complaints prompting patients to seek my help and one of the most complex conditions to treat. Fatigue is epidemic in this country: according to the Centers for Disease Control, between one and four million people in the United States have chronic fatigue syndrome (CFS). However, only 20 percent of these people are diagnosed. The number of people suffering is even larger when you consider all who "just" have chronic fatigue, but not CFS. The difference between chronic fatigue and CFS lies in the diagnostic criteria.

The CDC uses the 1994 CFS case definition, which requires meeting three criteria:

1. The individual has had severe chronic fatigue for six or more consecutive months, and the fatigue is not due to ongoing exertion or other medical conditions associated with fatigue. (These other conditions need to be ruled out by a doctor after diagnostic tests have been conducted.)

2. The fatigue significantly interferes with daily activities and work

3. The individual has four or more of the following eight symptoms concurrently:

   a. Post-exertion malaise (fatigue after you exert yourself) lasting more than 24 hours

   b. Unrefreshing sleep

    c. Significant impairment of short-term memory or concentration

    d. Muscle pain

    e. Pain in the joints without swelling or redness

    f. Headaches of a new type, pattern, or severity

    g. Tender lymph nodes in the neck or armpit

    h. A sore throat that is frequent or recurring

These symptoms should have persisted or recurred during six or more consecutive months of illness, and they cannot have first appeared before the fatigue.

But what about someone who has only three of the above symptoms? Or someone whose symptoms started three months ago? I diagnose these people with "chronic fatigue" (not CFS). They are suffering, and still need to be treated.

Unfortunately, those who suffer and are diagnosed with CFS are validated, but not cured. They feel relieved to have a diagnosis, but treatment options in conventional medicine are few. The rest of us with chronic fatigue push through our daily lives knowing something is wrong, but we are not sure what to do about it. There is a range from mild chronic fatigue to CFS, and I believe the total number afflicted today is probably closer to thirty million people in the United States.

Fortunately, in 2015, the United States Institute of Medicine renamed CFS as systemic exertion intolerance disease (SEID). The three symptoms they say must be present for diagnosis are impaired day-to-day functioning because of fatigue, malaise after exertion (physical, cognitive, or emotional), and unrefreshing sleep. The symptoms must also be accompanied by either cognitive impairment or orthostatic intolerance (low blood pressure), or both.

This is a much broader definition and much closer to my definition of chronic fatigue: a fatigue that persists over time and is not relieved by rest. In contrast, acute fatigue is fatigue that resolves with rest. In this book, anytime I mention fatigue, I am referring to chronic fatigue or SEID.

If you have fatigue with any of the symptoms listed above and it is compromising your quality of life, then *you* know you have chronic fatigue, and *I* know you have chronic fatigue. You don't need to be diagnosed with CFS/SEID to know you are suffering. The information presented in this book will support your recovery, regardless of where you are on the chronic fatigue spectrum. CFS/SEID is merely the more severe end of the fatigue spectrum.

No one would choose to have chronic fatigue, and any medical provider who believes that you are in their office for "no reason" is missing an opportunity for growth and compassion. Many of my patients have experienced emotional trauma from their interactions with conventional medical providers. This is because many medical providers feel shame when they can't help someone, and the feeling is so uncomfortable for them that they need to get that patient out of their office as soon as possible to relieve the discomfort. Unfortunately, they accomplish this by shaming the patient and causing emotional trauma.

So, once you realize you have chronic fatigue what do you do about it?

Why is it so Hard to Treat Fatigue?

If fatigue were caused by one thing, it would be pretty easy to treat. Like strep throat: you have a pain in your throat caused by an infection that resolves when treated with antibiotics. It's organized, simple, and logical. It fits our human thinking. But unfortunately, fatigue is not that simple.

Chronic fatigue has many different causes. Every person with fatigue has multiple causes, and these causes differ from person to person. One person's fatigue may be caused by chronic infections and adrenal dysfunction, and another person's fatigue may be caused by thyroid disease, mercury toxicity, and mold toxicity.

This is why it is so hard to treat. In conventional medicine, they believe there is no cause because they are only looking for a single cause. Research is largely unsuccessful because only one cause or treatment is tested at a time.

Additionally, when you are treating multiple causes, often you may treat several causes without an improvement in symptoms. This is because *all* of the causes need to be treated for the body to reach a state of balance and achieve symptom relief.

The way I describe it to my patients is that they have sixteen nails sticking out of the bottom of their foot, causing them pain. The more nails I remove, the less pain they will have, but they will still have pain until I remove all of them.

The Real Causes of Fatigue

To figure out the causes of your fatigue, we will be using your symptoms, physical signs, and laboratory testing. Once we find the causes, we can resolve them.

First, we need to make sure your fatigue is not resulting from a major medical illness like diabetes, cancer, or cardiovascular disease. Your personal medical provider can rule these out.

Once you've done so, it's time to move on to the most likely offenders.

I have organized this book into sections, based on what my clinical experience and research have revealed are the top causes of fatigue. These factors are summarized below, and we'll delve into each one in detail in the chapters that follow.

1. **Sleep**: Restorative sleep is essential for resolving fatigue. I will discuss the surprising causes of poor sleep and how to resolve them.

2. **Dehydration**: Most of us live in a state of chronic dehydration. Consuming enough water improves waste elimination and provides energy to the cells. I'll discuss the amount of water you should consume, when you should consume it, and how to make sure you're getting the cleanest water.

3. **Food toxins**: Foods can be good for you or bad for you, depending on how your immune system reacts to them. Food allergies and sensitivities can zap your energy and lead to fatigue. I know making changes to your diet is challenging; I will guide you through this process gently with lots of flexibility. I will discuss the food plan that I recommend to my patients and the one that I eat every day.

4. **Lack of exercise & movement**: Inadequate exercise and excess sitting play a significant role in fatigue and chronic disease today. Exercise elevates the mood and facilitates waste removal from the body. As humans, we need to move more—whether it's dancing, sports, or just taking the stairs. For people with fatigue, the last thing we want to do is exercise, and when we do, we suffer worse fatigue for days. So, we want to move our bodies only as much as we can without feeling

worse. I'll give you my favorite movement tips and when you shouldn't exercise.

5. **Emotional stress and trauma**: In today's busy world, mental and emotional stressors are all too common. Whether the stress is from our work or home lives, or from chronic, underlying emotional trauma like post-traumatic stress disorder (PTSD), or adverse childhood events (ACEs), there is a significant amount of emotional work that needs to be done to relieve these stressors. I have asked my wife and emotional stress expert Stacy S. Hirsch, MES, ACC, CDWF, to discuss this topic. She will discuss how to assess if you have had emotional trauma, how it affects your body, and what you can do to remedy it.

6. **Adrenal gland dysfunction**: The adrenal glands are small triangular glands that sit on top your kidneys and are responsible for producing cortisol. Cortisol is the hormone that regulates your response to stress, including mental, emotional, and physical stressors. Assessing your adrenal function is crucial for regulating circadian rhythm, sleep, blood sugars, blood pressure, and energy. We'll discuss the real causes of adrenal fatigue, how you can test for it, and how you can restore your adrenal glands to optimal function.

7. **Thyroid gland dysfunction**: Despite experiencing fatigue and other symptoms of low thyroid, patients are frequently told that their thyroid function is "normal." In reality, you probably have thyroid issues despite normal results on standard laboratory testing. I will discuss what tests to get, how to interpret them, what you need to do first, how to treat low thyroid, and even how to reverse your thyroid dysfunction.

8. **Sex hormone dysfunction**: Deficiencies or imbalances in progesterone, estrogen, and testosterone in men and women contribute to fatigue, and it's not just because you turned 50! I will teach you what you need to do to bring your body back into balance with or without taking prescription hormones.

9. **Nutrient deficiencies:** Deficiencies in iron, B12, folate, magnesium, and vitamin D are notorious for contributing to fatigue. I will discuss the laboratory tests you need to order, what the optimal range is for you, and how to replace any deficiencies correctly.

10. **Mitochondrial dysfunction**: The mitochondria are the energy centers of every cell in the body (except red blood cells). They are damaged by many other causes of fatigue: heavy metals, chemicals, molds, and infections. I will discuss how to get your mitochondria back on track and making energy again.

11. **Constipation**: If you're not stooling one to two times per day (preferably two), then you're constipated. When you're constipated, the toxins and waste products that you're trying to remove from your body are instead being reabsorbed through the large intestine and back into the bloodstream. This increases the toxic burden in your body and contributes to fatigue. I'll discuss the easy way to resolve this problem.

12. **Mold toxicity**: Half of all the buildings in our country have water damage, and most of those are growing mold. Mold toxicity is a huge problem for many of my patients. If your home has mold, you will not get better until you get it out of your environment

and your body. I'll tell you how to assess mold in your home and your body and how to remove it from both.

13. **Heavy metals, chemicals, and electromagnetic frequencies (EMFs)**: Today, toxic substances pollute our air, soil, food, and water. I will discuss the best ways to assess what toxins you may have in your body and how to remove them.

14. **Infections**: Infections from bacteria, spirochetes, parasites, viruses, fungi, and other microorganisms play a huge role in chronic fatigue. I'll discuss the art of assessing what infections you have, how to treat them, and what you need to do first.

It's only when we address each of these causes that we can be sure to resolve chronic fatigue.

The Fix Your Fatigue Program: A Four-Step Plan

I created the Fix Your Fatigue Program to resolve all of the causes of fatigue. It is a four-step plan that will:

1. Address the lifestyle foundations (sleep, food, movement, water, and emotions)

2. Replace deficiencies in nutrients and hormones

3. Remove toxicity caused by heavy metals, chemicals, molds, infections, EMFs, and stress

4. Repair emotions, lymph and detoxification pathways, mitochondria, organs, and the nervous system

Action Steps

1. Think about which causes you may have.

2. Join the conversation and share your story with people like you in our Fix Your Fatigue Facebook Group at fb.com/groups/fixyourfatigue.

3. Next step, let's start collecting some data to help you!

Chapter 2:
Fix Your Labs

"Don't guess, test" is a common refrain among medical practitioners, but it doesn't take into account the importance of the patient's symptoms. Some diagnoses can more easily be made based on clinical symptoms and some cannot. For example, symptoms associated with hormonal deficiencies, molds, and infections are a lot easier to identify from symptoms than those from heavy metals, chemicals, and nutrient deficiencies.

Consider these options for laboratory testing when assessing the causes of your fatigue:

1. Do all of the initial testing upfront so that you have all of the data.

2. Test the least expensive, most important tests first. Add in other testing as needed later.

3. Treat based on clinical symptoms; only add in testing when needed.

I prefer the second. Only order labs necessary for the diagnosis. I don't want you waste money on labs you don't need.

I will recommend lab tests I believe everyone should get for an overall health assessment. Then, only order the labs that I recommend if the symptoms and cases ring true for you and your condition.

Additionally, I will discuss throughout the book how to treat based on symptoms in addition to lab testing.

Where do I get a lab order?

You can acquire an order to do lab testing from your personal medical provider. If you don't have access to a medical provider who is able and willing to write the order for you, consider going through a third party like MyMedLab. MyMedLab sells you the laboratory tests that you want through their website. Once you have paid for the labs you want, you print out the order for the lab tests and take it to your local laboratory for the blood draw.

To assist you in this process, I setup a blood panel called the FYF Blood Panel to make it easier for you to order these labs at FYF.MyMedLab.com. I do not receive any compensation from this laboratory.

You want your blood to be drawn first thing in the morning (ideally before 9 a.m.) after you have fasted. Have nothing to eat and take no supplements or medications after midnight before the blood draw. Drink twenty ounces of water between the time you wake up and the blood draw. If it normally takes a phlebotomist several tries to draw enough blood, drink forty ounces of water mixed with one-quarter teaspoon of sea salt before the blood draw to make your blood vessels bigger and more stable.

In Appendix A, I have listed all of the lab tests that I discuss in this book and my recommendations for how you prioritize which ones to get. I have also included these in the chapters, so you won't need to keep referencing the appendix.

Here is the list of the top lab tests that I recommend you order now:

Blood testing:
(the FYF Blood Panel at FYF.MyMedLab.com)

- Thyroid Stimulation Hormone (TSH)
- Free T4
- Free T3
- Anti-thyroglobulin antibody
- Anti-thyroid peroxidase antibody
- Cortisol (not "free cortisol")
- DHEA-S
- Vitamin B12
- Folate
- Homocysteine
- 25 hydroxyvitamin D
- Magnesium
- Complete Metabolic Profile (CMP)
- TIBC
- Ferritin
- Complete Blood Count (CBC)
- Total testosterone
- Free testosterone

These tests will assess for most of the nutrient and hormonal deficiencies that cause fatigue.

The Plan

1. Go to FYF.MyMedLab.com and order the FYF Blood Panel or have the labs ordered by your personal medical provider.

2. Take the lab order to your local lab and have your labs drawn.

3. Give yourself a high five!

Now, let's get into the lifestyle changes that you can start while you are waiting for the labs to return.

Step I:
Lifestyle Foundations

Chapter 3:
Fix Your Sleep

*J*enny slept fine until her car accident. Suddenly, she had a hard time falling asleep and was up multiple times during the night. Her energy during the day decreased so dramatically that she had to take naps under her desk at work to get through the day. Her memory got worse, and she started losing her hair. The accident had stressed her adrenals and thyroid, upsetting her sleep and causing fatigue.

Background

Poor sleep is always a sign that something is wrong with the health of an individual. Sleep is a foundational requirement for good health, and sleep problems will nearly always contribute to fatigue. This may be from a lack of sleep or poor sleep quality—sleeping plenty of hours but awakening feeling tired and unrefreshed. You may have trouble falling asleep, staying asleep, getting deep, restorative sleep, or all the above. These problems are commonly referred to as insomnia.

It is estimated that between fifty and seventy million Americans suffer from sleep disorders—but the majority don't report sleep problems to their physicians, and most physicians don't take the time to inquire. The pervasive lack of appreciation for the importance of sleep has serious implications for public health.

Achieving seven to nine hours of deeply restorative sleep is a good goal, and sleeping less than seven is inadequate for most people. However, sleeping *more* than nine hours is also associated with poor health, so there seems to be a "sweet spot."

As humans, we should be awake during the day and asleep at night. Sleeping at night rejuvenates our bodies and minds and promotes healing. Being tired during the day and energized at night indicates a circadian rhythm dysfunction: your sleep cycle is out of sync! I will be discussing circadian rhythms in more detail in the next section.

Poor sleep interferes with nearly every biochemical process in the body. For example, while we sleep, our brain cells shrink by about 60 percent, which allows for more efficient waste removal. Sleep is also critical for balancing hormone levels, including melatonin. Melatonin is not just a "sleep hormone" but also an anti-cancer hormone, inhibiting the proliferation of a wide range of cancers. Poor sleep also inhibits leptin, the satiety ("I'm full") hormone.

Chronic sleep deprivation drives up inflammation, impairs blood sugar regulation, and raises the risk for many types of chronic disease. A study conducted by researchers at Harvard University found that inadequate sleep is associated with the following:

1. **Weight gain**: People sleeping less than six hours per night have higher body mass index. Poor sleep has been shown to cause increased insulin, decreased leptin (the satiety hormone), and increased ghrelin (the hunger hormone); inadequate sleep is now considered a risk factor for obesity and type 2 diabetes.

2. **Heart disease**: There is growing evidence of a connection between obstructive sleep apnea and heart disease; poor sleep has immediate detrimental effects on blood pressure as well.

3. **Mood disorders**: Chronic sleep issues are associated with depression, anxiety, and mental distress.

4. **Stress**: Poor sleep results in elevated cortisol levels.

5. **Shortened life expectancy**: Data from three large cross-sectional epidemiological studies revealed sleeping five hours or less per night increased the risk of death by roughly 15 percent.

Fascinating Sleep Facts

The following are taken from the National Sleep Foundation:

- One of the primary causes of excessive sleepiness among Americans is self-imposed sleep deprivation.

- Man is the only mammal that willingly delays sleep.

- Sleep disturbance generally worsens with increasing altitude, especially above 13,200 feet. This is thought to result from diminished oxygen levels and accompanying changes in respiration. Most people adjust to new altitudes in approximately two to three weeks.

- In general, exercising regularly makes it easier to fall asleep and contributes to sounder sleep. However, exercising sporadically or right before going to bed may make falling asleep more difficult.

- We naturally feel tired at two different times of the day: about 2 a.m. and 2 p.m. It is this natural dip in alertness that is primarily responsible for the post-lunch dip. *It can be exacerbated by adrenal dysfunction and a high carbohydrate meal at lunch.*

- The body NEVER adjusts to shift work. According to the International Classifications of Sleep Disorders, shift workers are at increased risk for a variety of chronic illnesses such as cardiovascular and gastrointestinal diseases and cancer.

- Thirty-six percent of Americans report being drowsy or falling asleep while driving.

- Rates of insomnia increase as a function of age, but most often the sleep disturbance is attributable to some other medical condition.

- There are individual differences in the need to nap, but in general, it's preferable to do your sleeping at night. The majority of people who nap in the afternoon are probably not sleeping enough at night or have adrenal dysfunction.

- Seasonal affective disorder (SAD) is believed to be influenced by the changing patterns of light and darkness that occur with the approach of winter.

Understanding Circadian Rhythms

Most people with sleep problems have a circadian rhythm dysfunction, which means their bodies don't know whether it's day or night. They're often sleepy during the day and wakeful at night.

Circadian rhythms are physical, mental, and behavioral changes that roughly follow a 24-hour cycle, primarily in response to environmental light and darkness. This is why it's so important to sleep in total darkness. Circadian rhythms are found in most living things, from humans to plants and even some microorganisms. Besides influencing sleep-wake cycles, they affect hormone release, body temperature, and other important functions. Abnormal circadian rhythms have been associated with sleep disorders, obesity, diabetes, and several types of mental illness.

Ari Whitten does a wonderful job of discussing this in more detail in his book and online program, The Energy Blueprint (theenergyblueprint.com).

Circadian rhythms and biological clocks are not the same things, but they are related—our circadian rhythms are driven by our biological clocks. Humans have a "master clock" that consists of a group of nerve cells in the brain (the suprachiasmatic nucleus), which controls the pineal gland's production of the "sleep hormone" melatonin. The best way to correct circadian rhythms is to retrain the body into a normal sleep pattern.

The Causes of Your Sleep Problems

To recreate your natural sleep rhythm, you need to address the causes. They are as follows:

1. Poor sleep habits (sleep hygiene)

2. Hormone imbalances (adrenal, thyroid, sex hormones)

3. Nutritional deficiencies (vitamin B12, vitamin D, iron, and magnesium)

4. Chronic infections (*Babesia*, *Bartonella*, and *Borrelia*)

Look familiar?

These causes of sleep issues are also some of the causes of chronic fatigue! Consequently, I will be addressing all of these as you go through the book.

You may be surprised to hear that besides changing sleep habits, I have more success getting people to sleep by supporting their adrenals, thyroid, vitamin B12, and iron in the *morning* than I do by giving them anything at night! This is because these hormonal and nutritional deficiencies affect the circadian rhythms.

At the beginning of this chapter, I talked about Jenny and how her sleep issues began after she had a car accident. This is because the stress of the car accident (both physically and emotionally) triggered a big release of cortisol from her adrenal glands. This release ended up depleting her adrenals and her thyroid and resulted in decreased energy and sleep problems.

In this chapter, we will be focusing on fixing your sleep hygiene and supporting your sleep with natural and pharmaceutical sleep aids.

Performing a Comprehensive Sleep Assessment

My basic approach to treating sleep problems is to identify and remove the cause. The first step is to perform a sleep inventory to identify potential issues related to sleep hygiene: the habits and practices that result in good sleep. I ask my patients a battery of questions, including the following:

- Do you go to bed after 11 p.m.?

- Do you get less than seven hours of sleep per night?

- Do you feel tired during the day and "wired" (have more energy) at night?

- Do you have a "monkey mind" where the stress of the day is keeping your brain going and preventing you from shutting it down?

- Do you startle easily?

- Do you go to bed and wake up at different times on weekdays than on weekends?

- Do you read or watch TV in bed?

- Do you discuss stimulating topics an hour or two before bedtime?

- Do you get into heated discussions late in the evening?

- Do you consume B vitamins, caffeine, or alcohol after dinner?

- Do you consume caffeine after 9 a.m.?

- Do you stay awake after 10 p.m., even after your body says it is time to sleep?

- Do you snore?

- Does your partner snore?

- Do you have pets or young children that awaken you during the night?

If the answer is "yes" to any of these, then there's a good chance your sleep quality may be significantly improved using sleep hygiene strategies.

Are You a Night Owl?

When your circadian rhythms are altered, you will feel more awake in the evenings. Additionally, most people will get a "second wind" after 11 p.m., leading them to accept the designation of a "night owl." Once you have fixed your circadian rhythms, this will no longer be the case, and you will find that your best hours for sleep are from 10 p.m. to 6 a.m.

Strategies for Improving Sleep

Implementing the following sleep strategies is the least expensive and most important thing you can do to improve your sleep.

1. **Sleep Window.** Your "sleep window" is the ideal time to go to sleep, and for most, it is between 9 and 10:30 p.m. It's helpful to go to bed during this window every night (even on the weekends) to consistently get seven to nine hours of sleep. If you get a "second wind"— the energy that keeps us awake after previously feeling tired – you know you've missed your sleep window.

   I have found that if you're not asleep by 10:30 p.m. on a consistent basis, you won't be able to resolve your fatigue.

2. **Sleep Cycles:** As adults, we have 1.5- or 2-hour sleep cycles while we sleep. This is the time that our sleep becomes lighter, and we transition into another phase of sleep. If you have a 1.5-hour sleep cycle, you will wake up feeling rested when you go to bed at 10:30 p.m. and wake up at 6 a.m. This is seven and a half hours of sleep in five 1.5-hour sleep cycles. If you have a 2-hour sleep cycle, you will wake up feeling rested when you sleep from 10 p.m. to 6 a.m. This is

eight hours of sleep in four 2-hour sleep cycles. Pay attention to how you feel after awakening from 1.5-hour sleep cycles versus 2-hour sleep cycles and adjust your sleep and wake times accordingly.

3. **Rise and Shine:** Go to bed and wake up at the same time every morning and evening, including weekends.

4. **Bedroom Activities:** The bedroom should be reserved for only sleep and sex. Reading and watching TV ideally should be done in a different room. However, some people can read in their bedrooms before bed without an issue.

5. **Napping:** Napping during the day is not ideal and is a sign that your circadian rhythms are off and your adrenal glands are compromised. If you feel the need to rest during the day, try to lie down without falling asleep and set a 15-minute timer. If you do need to nap during the day while we are fixing your adrenal glands, that's fine. Just know that it is temporary. You can gauge your progress based on your need to nap. My patients find that as their adrenal function improves, they no longer need to nap.

6. **Exercise:** Exercise can be beneficial for sleep. Some people sleep better when they exercise in the morning, whereas others sleep better exercising just before bed; experiment and do what works best for you.

7. **Foods:** Unstable blood sugar levels can interfere with sleep. Consuming protein every two to three hours during the day and right before bed can help prevent a blood sugar dip at night, which can trigger cortisol surges that delay sleep or awaken you during the

night. This is a great trick if you are waking between 1 a.m. and 3 a.m.

8. **Stimulants:** Reduce (or eliminate) overall caffeine intake, and refrain from consuming coffee and other caffeinated beverages after about 9 a.m. Caffeine can last up to twenty hours in the body! It also "whips" the adrenal glands into producing more cortisol, worsening adrenal fatigue. Chocolate in the afternoon and evening can also negatively affect sleep.

9. **Electronics:** Stop screen time one to two hours before bed. These devices emit blue light and trick the brain into thinking it is daytime. Get a blue light blocker for your computers and your phone. I recommend the app flux (flux.com) for your computer and Twilight for your Android phone and tablet. Many phones come with blue light blockers, but I find them inadequate. Your screen should have an orange hue.

10. **Lighting:** Your body knows what time it is based on its exposure to light. Make sure that your days are full of sunlight and your nights are absent of light. Sleep in complete darkness. This helps regulate the pineal gland, circadian rhythms, and melatonin production. If a nightlight is needed for navigation, install one with yellow, orange, or red light, as these wavelengths do not disrupt sleep (no blue light!). Salt lamps are wonderful for this purpose!

11. **Comfort:** Make sure your bed and your pillow are comfortable.

12. **Thermoregulation:** The body's heat regulation system is strongly linked to sleep cycles. Keeping the bedroom between 60 and 69 degrees F is

recommended. You want the body's core temperature to drop, but you don't want cold hands or feet, as that impairs blood flow and leads to restlessness. Taking a warm bath 90 to 120 minutes before bedtime is often helpful, so your core temperature is dropping about the time you fall asleep. Consider adding one or two cups of Epsom salt to the bath to get the relaxing effects of magnesium.

13. **Stress:** Develop a relaxing bedtime routine. Create a stress-free environment after dinner, which means no arguing or watching scary movies. If you are experiencing stress, find a counselor or health coach knowledgeable in Mindfulness-Based Stress Reduction (MBSR) techniques, or an Emotional Freedom Techniques (EFT) practitioner. The MBSR course can be done online.

14. **Pets:** If pets interrupt your sleep, keep them out of the bedroom at night. Your animals will adjust, and so will you—your sleep is THAT important!

15. **EMFs:** Be mindful about electromagnetic fields (EMFs) in the bedroom, which can disrupt the pineal gland and its melatonin production. Ideally, turn off wireless routers, computers, and cell phones for the night. Even the electrical panels (fuses) that control the bedroom can be shut down at night to reduce electrical background "noise."

16. **When to Get Out of Bed:** If you can't sleep, staying in bed can be frustrating and typically raises anxiety. Instead, after thirty minutes of not sleeping, get up, turn the lights on low (or not at all), listen to soft music or read a book, and then return to bed when you feel sleepy. If you're reading a book on your

phone, make sure you have a blue light blocker turned on.

17. **Snoring or Morning Headaches:** If you snore or experience morning headaches, consider getting a sleep study to rule out sleep apnea. If apnea is confirmed, ask your doctor about a dental appliance, Breath Right nasal strips, or a CPAP machine to improve the flow of oxygen during sleep. Low oxygen levels at night and increased pressure from snoring will decrease the quality of sleep and can lead to other medical issues such as high blood pressure, headaches, and lung and heart problems. Chronic sinus problems can also play a role and should be evaluated.

Menopause and Sleep

If you're forty-five to fifty-five years old and have just started having sleep problems (and never had them before), then your sleep issues are probably from menopause and sex hormone deficiencies. Other signs include vaginal dryness, anxiety, dry hair, and hair loss.

Progesterone helps women fall asleep, and estrogen helps them stay asleep. So, if you are having trouble falling asleep, you may need to take progesterone. If you are having a hard time staying asleep, then you may need to take estrogen.

You can replace your estrogen, progesterone, and testosterone in accordance with my recommendations in the Fix Your Sex Hormones chapter.

Infections and Sleep

Certain infections are active at night and can disrupt your sleep. The most common culprits are those that can get into your nervous system and affect your ability to relax. They can also cause nutritional and hormonal deficiencies, exacerbating your sleep problems. In my practice, I see primarily *Bartonella*, *Babesia*, and *Borrelia*. You can learn more about how to treat these in the Fix Your Stealth Infections chapter.

Sleep Aids

I once heard Joe Burrascano, MD, a Lyme disease expert, say, "I don't care if you hit your patients over the head with a hammer; you must get them to sleep. If they don't sleep, they can't heal." So, while we are working on the causes of your sleep issues, I also want to give you a sleep aid in the meantime. As always, natural therapies are best as long as they work.

I recommend starting with botanicals (herbs), nutrients, and neurotransmitter precursors that help people fall asleep and stay asleep during the night. These supplements will help your body recreate its circadian rhythm. The ones that I recommend include:

- Magnesium, a wonderfully relaxing mineral that promotes sleep.

- Phosphatidylserine to decrease adrenal stress and shut off the "monkey mind."

- Melatonin, a multifunctional hormone whose main role lies in its involvement in the control of the circadian rhythms. Melatonin mediates the body's response to variations in natural light. Darkness into the eye tells the brain to make melatonin so the body can prepare for sleep mode. Its production should peak at night, and it is instrumental in maintaining quality sleep patterns.

- GABA. Gamma-amino butyric acid, the central nervous system "relaxer." This amino acid allows your nervous system to calm down.

- German chamomile binds to receptors in the central nervous system and decreases anxiety.

- Valerian root has demonstrated sedative effects due to its ability to induce the release of GABA from brain tissue.

- Passionflower reduces anxiety and promotes sleep.

- Lemon balm has been suggested to improve calmness via the relaxing action of GABA.

- L-theanine has been clinically proven to reduce stress and improve the quality of sleep.

- 5-HTP can be used in conjunction with melatonin as a precursor to serotonin, which can further support melatonin production during the night to help with staying asleep.

- Cannabis has many medicinal properties, including anti-anxiety and sedation. If you can obtain it legally, tell the dispensary that you want an "indica strain that is high in CBDs." I recommend making a cannabis infusion in olive oil.

You don't have to take all of these separately. Below I recommend products that combine many of these for a synergistic effect.

Pharmaceutical Sleep Aids

If the natural therapies aren't working and you need to go to the next step, I recommend the prescription Trazodone. It was developed as an anti-depressant but is better as a sleep aid. Side effects are minimal but include constipation, sedation, and low blood pressure.

Other options include Ambien, Klonopin, Sonata, and Lunesta, but I only use them if everything else doesn't work because of their addictive potential.

Summary

Addressing sleep issues is foundational for good health, whether or not you suffer from fatigue. The strategies in this chapter can be used by anyone whose goal is optimal health. That said, changing your lifestyle and behavior requires energy. If you are battling severe fatigue, achieving restorative sleep is essential before moving on to address other potential issues that require greater effort, such as changing your diet or exercise.

Sleep problems affect a large proportion of the U.S. population and are a serious contributor to many chronic illnesses, including obesity, type 2 diabetes, heart disease, and mental illness. Poor sleep increases inflammation, drives up cortisol levels, and wreaks overall havoc with hormones and metabolism. Sleep problems range from simply not getting enough sleep to experiencing poor quality, non-restorative sleep. Patients typically underreport sleep problems to their doctors, and doctors typically neglect to inquire.

My approach to treating sleep problems is to identify and remove the causes. These include poor sleep hygiene, nutritional and hormonal deficiencies, and chronic infections.

Most people with poor sleep have circadian rhythm dysfunction. An important first step is assessing sleep hygiene: the habits and practices that set the stage for optimal sleep. Lifestyle factors such as diet, exercise, stress, family dynamics, evening activities, screen time, and overall sleep environment are important considerations when evaluating and treating sleep problems and fatigue. Snoring and sleep apnea must also be evaluated and addressed.

Testing and treating any nutrient deficiencies, hormone imbalances, and infections are necessary.

While treating the causes, natural and pharmaceutical sleep aids may need to be utilized.

The Plan

If you're having problems sleeping, here's how to get your sleep back on track.

Start implementing the sleep hygiene strategies above. Choose one at a time if it feels overwhelming to implement more than that. The most important ones are:

1. Going to bed at 10 p.m. in a dark room, away from your electronics.

2. Relaxing after dinner with low-stress activities.

3. Avoiding caffeine (coffee and even chocolate) to see if that makes a difference in your sleep.

4. Order your labs if you haven't done so already so you can find out if you have any deficiencies in hormones and nutrients that might be affecting your sleep. I will discuss replacing any deficiencies in the subsequent chapters.

5. Start re-creating your circadian rhythms with natural sleep aids:

6. Start Insomnitol 2 caps/night. If you are groggy in the morning, decrease to 1 cap per night. This product has most of the natural sleep aids previously discussed.

7. Start magnesium chelate 1 capsule per night.

8. Start taking a magnesium bath every night. Use Epsom salt 2 cups or Magnegel (magnesium gel) 1 tsp in hot water for 30 minutes.

9. Start Phosphatidylserine 1 cap/night

10. If you snore, get a sleep study to rule out obstructive sleep apnea. You'll need a referral from your medical provider.

11. If your sleep is not improving, then start trazodone 25mg/night and increase by 25mg every three nights until you are sleeping through the night or you reach a maximum of 200mg/night. Your medical provider must prescribe this. Once you have treated the causes and you are sleeping well, you can wean off of this by 25mg every week.

12. If your sleep has been worse since menopause, you probably are deficient in progesterone and estrogen.

See the Fix Your Sex Hormones chapter for more information.

13. Once your sleep hygiene and deficiencies are remedied, if your sleep is still not ideal, then address *Bartonella*, *Babesia*, and *Borrelia* with the recommendations I make in the chapter on infections.

Action Steps

1. Implement one or two sleep hygiene strategies.

2. Order the new supplements discussed in this chapter. You can find them under the Sleep Support category in our online store here: us.fullscript.com/welcome/drhirsch

3. Add your new sleep supplements to your Treatment Schedule & Calendar (free in the member area at fixyourfatigue.org/members.)

4. Set alarms on your phone to remind you to take your supplements.

5. Track your sleep symptoms on your Symptom Calendar (free in the member area).

6. Questions? Ask people in our Facebook group (fb.com/groups/fixyourfatigue) questions like these:

   a. *Which sleep strategy helped your sleep the most?*

   b. *Which natural sleep aid helped your sleep the most?*

   c. *What is your favorite blue light blocker for your phone and computer?*

7. Get excited to Fix Your Water in the next chapter!

Chapter 4:
Fix Your Water

*J*ohn *didn't like to drink water. He hated the lack of taste and preferred juice instead. Unfortunately, he was starting to get fatigued and began putting on weight and urinating all the time. It was only when he stopped drinking juice and started drinking four liters of water per day that his symptoms resolved. He was amazed!*

Background

The foundation for a healthy life at its most basic level includes putting the right stuff into your body and taking the bad stuff out.

A healthy body relies on the following:

1. **Nutrients**: The right nutrients to run all of the biochemical pathways necessary for life and function in each of the cells in our bodies.

2. **Water**: Clean water for cellular function and to remove waste products from the body.

3. **Movement**: Physical movement to produce energy and remove waste products through the lymph and excretory systems.

You can see how your food choices, the amount of water that you drink, and the amount and type of movement that you do each day do more than just relieve hunger and thirst and maintain a stable weight!

In the next few chapters, I will discuss the foundational lifestyle habits to adopt to improve your fatigue.

At the end Step I, I will give you a backstage pass to the daily habits I have implemented to be successful in resolving my chronic fatigue.

Dehydration

Dehydration is incredibly common. In fact, 75 percent of Americans may suffer from chronic dehydration and don't know it. Eighty percent of our body weight is made up of water, and 99 percent of the molecules in our body are water molecules! Consuming enough water improves waste elimination and provides energy to our cells. Consequently, our health and energy are very dependent on the amount of water we consume.

Testing

You can tell if you're dehydrated based on laboratory work (looking at your kidneys) and physical exam (looking at your skin). On your blood tests, you can look at the health of your kidneys by looking at your blood urea nitrogen (BUN), creatinine (Cr) and Cystatin C levels. If your BUN:Cr ratio is above 20, or if your Cr or cystatin C is elevated, then you may be dehydrated, and your kidneys are not happy because they are not getting enough water and blood to filter them. Sometimes, however, your kidneys may not be happy, and you may appear dehydrated because your body is not holding on to the water you are consuming.

When someone is dehydrated, they usually lose water out of their skin, and the skin becomes less elastic. Consequently, when you pinch dehydrated skin, it will stay in that position and slowly resolve. If the skin is not dehydrated, it should be more elastic and return to normal immediately.

You can also "test" your hydration status by the color of your urine. If your urine is clear, you are hydrated. If it is yellow, you are dehydrated. The darker yellow it is, the more dehydrated you are.

The Plan

1. Start drinking half of your body weight in ounces of water every day throughout the day. For example, if you weigh 140 pounds, you should drink 70 ounces of water every day. However, if you have adrenal issues (see the Fix Your Adrenals chapter), you will need to drink 25 percent more water per day (or approximately 90 ounces for a 140-pound person). Most people need three to four liters per day. A liter is approximately a quart or 32 ounces. Keep increasing your water intake until your urine is no longer yellow.

2. Start drinking one-half to one liter upon waking and 30 minutes before each meal. Be aware that if you drink water with meals or too close to mealtime, it can dilute the digestive juices in your stomach and intestines and affect your digestion.

3. Start adding a pinch of natural sea salt (Celtic or Himalayan sea salt – NOT table salt) to each glass/container of water. This is great for your adrenals (more on this in the Fix Your Adrenals chapter) and your kidneys and helps you hold on to the water and stay hydrated.

4. Consider drinking more coconut water. Coconut water is an excellent natural electrolyte-balancing beverage but is high in sugar, so use it in moderation, such as during a workout. Stay away from commercially prepared so-called "energy drinks."

5. Consider filtering your water with a countertop or whole house water filter by Aquasana.com.

Action Steps

1. Decide what water bottle you're going to use. Consider glass and stainless steel to avoid plastic (toxic). I like klean kanteen.

2. Decide how much and what times of day you are going to drink water. (i.e. 20 ounces when you first wake up, 30 minutes before meals, and 1 hour before bed)

3. Then, add your new water routine to your Treatment Schedule. This will help you keep track of it and make sure it gets done!

4. Set a "drink water" appointment on your phone's calendar to remind you to drink water. When the reminder goes off, stop everything and drink 15-30 ounces. Chugging is okay!

5. Track your symptoms on the Symptom Calendar and see how they improve with drinking more water.

6. Questions? Ask people in the Facebook group questions like these:

   a. *What is your favorite water bottle?*

   b. *What is your favorite kind of sea salt?*

   c. *Do you use a water filter? Which one?*

7. Continue to implement the lifestyle changes you have made thus far.

8. Continue eating more meat and vegetables and avoiding grains and sugars.

9. Get excited to Fix Your Food in the next chapter!

Chapter 5:
Fix Your Food

The doctor injected my ear with a numbing medicine. "This will sting a little," he said. I was fifteen years old. A minute later I felt him tugging on my ear, and then he presented to me the cyst he had pulled out of my earlobe. It wasn't my first one. I had acne that formed into cysts. "Is there anything I can do to prevent this from happening again?" I asked him. "No," he said. "It just happens." It wasn't until ten years later, after prolonged courses of antibiotics and prescription Accutane (toxic levels of vitamin A) that I eliminated dairy from my diet and resolved my cystic acne.

Background

Food is a touchy subject, especially if you're not feeling well. We have a lot of emotional attachments to it, and it can give us joy at times when nothing else can. This is why I'm going to make some recommendations that you can implement gradually.

I thought about waiting until later in the book to discuss proper food choices and food allergies, but I realized that would be a disservice to you. You see, the improvements I have seen in the health of my patients when they change their food choices are amazing. In fact, I used to require everyone to go through the food elimination diet to figure out what food allergies they had before I would even take them on as patients. This is because food allergies play a significant role as a cause and contributor to fatigue.

The first step in the process of making better food choices is to move toward a Paleo diet and eliminate gluten.

The next step is to determine which foods may be making you sick (food allergies) and remove them from your diet.

Before we start this process, I want to be clear about something. Do not change your diet if it is going to stress you out. If you notice this happening, do not change your diet. Just move on to the next chapter. If you can eliminate only gluten right now, that is a huge victory. If not, no worries. You can come back to this when you have more energy. Baby steps!

The Paleolithic Food Plan

Regardless of your state of health, I believe the Paleo diet (or food plan) is the best dietary approach for optimal health and longevity. The Paleo food plan consists primarily of meat, vegetables, nuts, and seeds, with low amounts of fruit and sugar, and no grains. It is the food plan I recommend to all of my patients and the one that I live by every day.

No grains?! But why? (you may be asking). Let me tell you the story of gluten, the main protein found in wheat.

The Story of Gluten

Gluten and gliadin are proteins that cause much of the inflammation and problems associated with the consumption of wheat products. The word gluten literally means "glue" in Latin. In ancient times, a concoction of wheat flour plus water was used for plaster. Even today, wheat plays a role in industrial adhesives (paints, paper mache, and bookbinding glue). A high number of disulfide bonds (sulfur-to-sulfur) gives gluten its adhesive properties.

If you're wondering if eating a food that makes excellent glue might NOT be great for your digestive tract, then you're onto something!

Humans in our present form have been around for about three million years. Wheat has only been around for about ten thousand—and we're just not equipped to consume it.

Unfortunately, wheat grown in this country is not healthy, even non-GMO wheat. Selective breeding and hybridization have turned modern wheat into a product that's foreign to the human body. Upon digestion, modern wheat breaks down into a massive number of proteins, each with a distinct potential for stimulating the production of antibodies and autoimmunity.

Common wheat bread (*Triticum aestivum*) has been associated with more than 23,788 proteins thus far. In fact, the genome for common wheat bread is actually 6.5 times larger than the human genome! I tell my patients that eating wheat is like eating a sock. Our body sees it as foreign and tries to attack it and get rid of it.

Rising rates of celiac disease are merely the tip of the iceberg. In his article "The Dark Side of Wheat—New Perspectives on Celiac Disease and Wheat Intolerance," Sayer Ji suggests that celiac disease be viewed not as an unhealthy response to a healthy food, but as a healthy response to an unhealthy food. He suggests we see the symptoms of celiac disease as "expressions of bodily intelligence, rather than deviance." He goes on to write:

People with celiac disease may have an advantage over the apparently non-afflicted because those who are "non-symptomatic" and whose wheat intolerance goes undiagnosed or misdiagnosed because they lack the classic symptoms may suffer in ways that are equally or more damaging, but expressed more subtly.

So, why does Western society consume so much wheat? Because it's so addictive... *literally*.

During digestion, glutenous grains can break down into gluteomorphins. Gluteomorphins (yes, that does say morphine!) are food opioids, able to travel through the bloodstream to your brain and bind to opioid receptors. This is why wheat is physiologically addictive, and eliminating consumption of wheat products can produce symptoms of withdrawal, akin to discontinuing a narcotic, albeit much milder.

William Davis, MD, has written an excellent book, *Wheat Belly*. He details our history with gluten and the consequences of consuming it - leaky gut, inflammation, food allergies, and autoimmunity. Gluten damages your intestines *every* time you consume it whether you are overtly reacting to it or not. So, I recommend that *everyone* avoid it.

Dairy is also a food opioid, with caseomorphins representing 80 to 90 percent of the protein fragments produced from the digestion of cow's milk.

Sugar may be the worst! Sugar scientist Dr. Robert Lustig explains that sugar is highly addictive, lighting up the reward centers of your brain like a fireworks display, similar to cocaine and nicotine.

All of these foods highjack your brain by altering its chemistry and fueling cravings and compulsions to overeat. It's no wonder sugar and wheat are the little darlings of the processed food industry.

What foods contain gluten?

Gluten is mainly found in grains; however, it can also be found hidden in dairy products, cosmetics, and processed foods. For our purposes, I am going to focus on the grains.

The following grains contain gluten: Wheat, barley, spelt, kamut, rye, triticale and oats.

The following grains DO NOT contain gluten: White and brown rice, corn, gluten-free oats, millet, quinoa, amaranth, teff, tapioca, and buckwheat.

Corn Gluten

Yes, I just said that corn is gluten-free. However, new research is emerging to the contrary. The proteins in corn (sometimes referred to as "corn gluten") can actually mimic those in gluten and cause similar symptoms and problems. I definitely consider the removal of corn from the diet when I'm not seeing the improvement in health that I anticipate.

Weight Gain and Gluten

Consuming gluten causes water retention (like most food allergies) and consequently weight gain.

When people go on the Paleo food plan and stop consuming gluten, they usually lose ten percent of their body weight in the first two months and continue to lose three pounds per month until they get down to a healthy weight. Some people even get down to the weight they were in high school! (As long as they were healthy in high school). Please note, however, if you have many of the toxin causes of fatigue, you may have a harder time getting down to your goal weight.

Balancing Your Blood Sugar

Besides removing gluten and moving toward the Paleo food plan, you're also going to want to eat at regular intervals throughout the day. This is a great way to keep your energy steady during the day and prevent any mid-morning and mid-afternoon energy "crashes."

Regulating your blood sugar is best accomplished by consuming protein and fat every three hours. Fruit, nuts, seeds, and meat bars (EPIC bars, Tanka Bites) make great snacks. I recommend the following schedule:

- Breakfast at 7 a.m.

- Snack at 10 a.m.

- Large lunch at noon

- Snack at 3 p.m.

- Small dinner at 6 p.m.

Food Allergies

Food allergies can cause almost any symptom the body can manifest, including fatigue. The gastrointestinal tract maintains a delicate balance of good bacteria, specialized immune cells, and various neurological and hormonal activities. In fact, 80 percent of your immune system resides in your gut, so anything you put in your mouth can trigger a reaction. Once your digestive system detects what it considers a "foreign particle," your immune system reacts, and the inflammation that follows creates pain and dysfunction.

The Causes of Food Allergies

There are several reasons why people develop food allergies. They are caused by a "total body burden" of things that are not supposed to be in the body. The immune system becomes activated by an overabundance of heavy metals, chemicals, molds, infections, other allergies, and emotions. I call them the *usual suspects* and will be referring to them as such throughout the book.

Once activated, your immune system can become overly reactive to foods, particularly hybridized and modified foods. These are foods that have been processed, and our body recognizes them as "foreign" and not from nature. They can damage the lining of your gastrointestinal tract, permitting food particles to trigger an immune response through a condition called "leaky gut."

To decrease the inflammation caused by this process, you need to remove the problem foods. For many people, this makes a big difference in their energy, but for others, not so much. For these folks, more of the "total body burden" has to be removed before they will have success. Then removing the food allergies results in improved energy.

So, once you figure out which foods are toxic for you, do you need to eliminate them for the rest of your life?

No. It turns out that when you get rid of the *usual suspects* from your body (and decrease your "total body burden"), the immune system relaxes and ceases to react as strongly and frequently to foods. You just have to be smart and consume these foods infrequently or as frequently as you can "get away with" before inflammation is triggered. Conversely, if you feel so good off these foods that you never want to eat them again, that's okay too. You may also find that as you learn more about why some of these foods are bad, you may choose not to consume them even if you don't react to them. This is ideal.

Leaky Gut Syndrome

The term "leaky gut syndrome" describes increased intestinal permeability. The intestinal lining has become overly porous. It no longer serves as an effective barrier to the rest of your body—that is, it begins to "leak."

Your intestine, or gut, is the first line of defense against foreign particles, pathogenic (disease-causing) bacteria, and other invaders. Its lining contains closely spaced microvilli designed to absorb properly digested nutrients from foods and transport them across mucosal cells into your bloodstream. Your body relies on this screening process to get crucial nutrients *in* and keep unwanted particles *out*.

Drugs, environmental toxins, stress, certain foods, and other things can damage your gut lining and microvilli. Holes formed in the gut wall allow these larger undigested particles to cross into your bloodstream. Once there, your body sees them as dangerous invaders and goes on the offense—and system-wide inflammation ensues. Before you know it, the body produces antibodies, and you have food allergies and sensitivities.

So, the foods themselves are not the problem—it's the body's reaction to them. People can experience adverse reactions to ordinarily healthy foods, as well as reactions to unhealthy ones.

The Food Elimination Diet

To reduce the overall burden on the immune system, you must decrease inflammation by removing the foods that are triggering the reaction. This is most easily done with a food elimination diet. You cannot resolve your fatigue if you are eating foods that are making you sick. The eliminated foods can be reintroduced later, once the body has been desensitized.

To figure out which foods are a problem for you, you need to remove the most problematic foods for twenty-one days, reintroduce them, and see how your body reacts. After twenty-one days, your immune system is less reactive, since it no longer sees these foreign food particles that aren't supposed to be present. It does, however, still "remember" the foods that were causing your symptoms. Consequently, when you reintroduce a food that is a problem for you, your immune system will attack the food and cause inflammation, and your symptoms will return.

I recommend that you add one food back into your diet every four days, and watch for reactions. Your immune system may react to a food immediately after consumption or up to four days afterward. This is why we choose four days in between food introductions.

The top eleven food allergens are the following:

1. Gluten-containing grains

2. Dairy

3. Eggs

4. Soy

5. Corn

6. Coffee

7. Chocolate

8. Alcohol

9. Sugar

10. Peanuts

11. Oranges

The most common culprit is gluten, followed by dairy. I cannot emphasize how important it is to remove both of these if you suffer from fatigue. If you can only remove one food, make it gluten.

When reintroducing foods, you will add back one type of food at a time and consume it two to three times per day for three days. This is called the Oral Food Challenge Test (OFCT). Carefully monitor your reactions. You need *three full days* for each food type to learn whether or not your immune system is reacting. Ninety-five percent of the time your body will react to a food allergy in the first three days.

I recommend that you start with the bottom of the list first (the less problematic foods) as you add foods back in. For example, add in citrus on day twenty-two and eat it three times per day for three days, then add in peanuts the same way and so on.

For groups of food like dairy, add in one section of the group at a time. For example, add in cheese on the first day and eat it liberally for the first three days. Have a cheese party! Then on day four, try yogurt. Four days after that, test milk, and then ice cream, etc. Get as specific as you want—for example, test cheddar, Swiss, and goat cheese separately—and pay attention to how you feel after each. If you develop symptoms, then stop the food causing the reaction and stay on the diet until the symptoms resolve. Then you can start testing again. The reactive food then goes to the local food bank as a donation. Getting it out of the house reduces temptation!

You would follow the same principles for testing gluten and grains. For example, you might not react to spelt, but you could react to barley or rye, so each should be tested separately. Research shows that gluten can stay in your body and trigger an immune response for up to six months (after one bite!), so I recommend staying off gluten for at least three months (though even three months may not be sufficient). For my patients with fatigue, I recommend staying away from gluten altogether for reasons I'll be addressing next.

If you can only remove one food per month, that's fine! Remove it for twenty-one days, then add it back in and see how you feel. If you do not react, then remove the next food for the next month.

I also highly recommend that everyone in your household go through this process with you. Parents generally see improvement in their children's behaviors, acne, digestive symptoms, sleep, and mood. It can make a huge difference in their lives!

Testing for Food Allergies

Since the food elimination diet is hard work, patients ask me about other food allergy testing that may be available. These are usually blood tests and generally test for the immune system's reaction to foods. They test for the IgG immunoglobulin or inflammatory markers. Unfortunately, I have not found them to be particularly accurate, so I do not recommend them unless we know there is a reaction to a food, but we can't figure out which. The reality is that as you remove the *usual suspects* from your immune system, you become less reactive to foods, and the results of these tests would change often during your treatment. Stick with the food elimination diet and the oral food challenge test. They're the gold standard, and you're worth it!

After the Food Elimination Diet, What Comes Next?

If you implement a food elimination diet but don't notice a significant difference in your symptoms, it doesn't necessarily mean the diet is not beneficial. As already discussed, you may have a lot of the *usual suspects* to remove. Diet is just one piece of the puzzle—a critical piece.

Let's say your foot has twenty nails (representing the causes of your fatigue) causing inflammation (pain and dysfunction). If you remove just one nail (food allergies), it may not make a difference in how you feel even though you are decreasing the inflammation a bit. The total inflammation may be too high for you to notice the difference. You may need to remove a significant number of the nails (fatigue causes) before you experience an improvement in your symptoms. Make sense?

With some of my patients, such as those with chronic pain, I recommend a food elimination diet for a substantial length of time, *without* challenging the foods back in. This is because we need to decrease the inflammation and give the body every possible chance of recovery and remove every possible immune trigger. It's is a great strategy for just about everyone.

If you don't see any improvement with the diet, and it's too stressful to continue on it without seeing improvement, then stop it for now and come back to it in six months. If you can at least eliminate gluten (and even better, gluten and dairy!), you have a great start in making a big difference in decreasing your inflammation and resolving your fatigue.

After the elimination diet, I transition my patients to the Paleo diet as previously discussed. In its simplest form, it is meat and vegetables. Just focus on that, and you'll do fine. A basic rule that you can use is that when you sit down to eat, half of your plate should be made up of vegetables, one-quarter meat, and one-quarter starchy vegetable. I know that sounds like a lot, but eating plenty of vegetables gives you the vitamins, minerals, enzymes, and insoluble fiber that you need for lasting energy.

Don't Stress...

Yes, I know I've said it a few times in this chapter, but I'm going to say it again...

Changing your diet may be the most challenging aspect of fixing your fatigue. It is something you can do on your own, without investing in supplements or doctor visits. But for many, giving up an addictive food substance like sugar, wheat, or dairy only adds stress and contributes to exhaustion.

Please don't stress over your diet. I don't want this part of the program to cause you to quit it all together. Go easy on yourself. Make these changes in small stages if you're up for it. Or come back to this later.

A reasonable first step can be replacing all of the gluten products in your home with gluten-free products. Just watch the sugar content of these products!

Summary

Food allergies can be a factor in fatigue. Eighty percent of your immune system resides in your gut, so anything you put into your mouth can trigger a reaction. Once your body sees what it thinks is a "foreign particle," your immune system reacts, and inflammation can result, which presents with a variety of symptoms including fatigue.

Most food allergies occur when your immune system is overburdened with the *usual suspects*: heavy metals, chemicals, molds, infections, allergies, electromagnetic frequencies, and emotions.

Increased intestinal permeability, or "leaky gut syndrome," can also result in food allergies and sensitivities. Undigested particles pass through your intestinal wall and into your bloodstream, where they trigger an immune response.

The best way to treat food allergies is with a food elimination diet. Eliminated foods can be gradually reintroduced once symptoms have resolved. Gluten and dairy are typically the worst offenders. Excess sugar is also very inflammatory and places a tremendous strain on the immune system.

The Paleo diet is an excellent eating plan after completing the food elimination diet.

The Plan

1. Start eating more meat and vegetables and avoiding grains and sugars. Half of your plate should be vegetables at every meal.

2. Start replacing all of the gluten products in your home with gluten-free products. Watch the sugar content of these products.

3. Learn more about the Paleo diet from the handout by Valerie Burke, MSN, in the member area.

4. Purchase Paleo snack food to have at work and home when you get hungry and every three hours. I like Tanka Bites, EPIC bars, seeds, nuts, and fresh fruit.

Action Steps

1. Want to get the food elimination diet, meal plans, and shopping list handouts that I recommend to my patients? Login to our free membership site at fixyourfatigue.org/members and download the food elimination diet handout.

2. Set alarms on your phone to remind you to eat throughout the day.

3. Track your symptoms on your Symptom Calendar (handout in the member area) when reintroducing foods that you have eliminated on the food elimination diet.

4. Questions? Ask people in our Facebook group (fb.com/groups/fixyourfatigue) questions like these:

    a. *Which foods did you react to the most?*

    b. *What are the best gluten-free breads?*

    c. *Anyone have a good Paleo muffin recipe?*

    d. *What is your favorite Paleo dessert/breakfast?*

5. Congratulations on completing another chapter! Way to go!

6. In the next chapter, we are going to Fix Your Movement!

Chapter 6:
Fix Your Movement

I had achieved a level of energy that I hadn't had in ten years. My energy was an 8 out of 10. I felt good, but I wasn't back to my old self yet. My body wanted to move, dance, and jump. I found myself jumping in place until my calves hurt. The energy was increasing in my cells, and my body was responding. I found that when I introduced regular exercise into my life, my energy increased even more.

Background

Inadequate exercise and excessive sitting play a significant role in fatigue and chronic disease today. I tell my patients that sitting is the new smoking! Numerous recent studies have shown excessive sitting may shorten your lifespan—*even among those who faithfully go to the gym!* So, if your activities are limited to walking from your cubicle to your car and then to your couch each day, you are inviting myriad health problems, only one of which is chronic fatigue.

The good news is that increased movement has been scientifically shown to help reduce the symptoms of fatigue. In one study, 75 percent of chronic fatigue patients who were able to engage in exercise—particularly aerobic exercise—reported increased fitness, decreased fatigue, and improved daily functioning after one year.

That said, be sure you're administering "the correct dose" of exercise because overdoing it can impede your progress. You will know if you're over-exercising if you feel worse afterward or the next day. If you do feel worse, then cut back, because pushing too hard can drain your adrenal glands of cortisol.

Exercise elevates the mood and improves detoxification. As humans, we need to move more—whether it's dancing, sports, or just taking the stairs. What fun movement do you like to do? Every culture incorporates some form of movement because of its importance for health and mood. So get moving!

I recommend a little exercise every day to start. If you need recovery time, go to every other day. Set a schedule, put it on your calendar, and stick to it!

Testing

To determine how much exercise you can do without draining your adrenals, start by doing five jumping jacks each day and increase by one jumping jack a day until you feel worse after you exercise. Switch up your routine with different exercises if your body doesn't respond well to one or the other. Consider pushups, sit-ups, burpees, squats, and plank pose.

Treatment

1. **Move, move, move!** Engage in a little more movement every day. Start small. For example, just ten jumping jacks or dancing around your living room every day can produce a noticeable difference. I've included a few ideas below, and I'm sure you will think of others.

2. **Fitness trackers**: Fitness trackers can be helpful reminders about your daily activity—or lack thereof. Experts recommend 7,000 to 10,000 steps per day, *but again, start small.* Maybe you need to start with a goal of 1,000 steps or even fewer in the beginning.

Make it an achievable goal, and ramp up as your health and activity tolerance improve.

3. **Fitness apps**: There are some great fitness apps available today, and many are free. Consider trying a seven-minute workout app for some interval training.

4. **Walking:** Don't underestimate the benefits of walking. There are daily opportunities to increase your steps. Walk your dog, "walk" your child, park farther away, walk on your lunch hour, and take the stairs.

5. **Hoops**: For you basketball fans, shoot a few hoops after work. Make it fun!

6. **Exercise groups**: Yoga, Pilates, and Tai Chi are powerful yet gentle forms of movement that are adaptable to any fitness level and will build your social support system as well. Having a class to go to can also help with accountability.

7. **Burpees**: Burpees can be done in your living room or office without any equipment—all you need is your body. They involve standing, squatting, and some variation of a push-up. There are many versions, and they can be adapted to just about any fitness level. YouTube "burpees for beginners.

8. **Rebounders**: Rebounders are mini-trampolines upon which you can bounce or jog. They are small enough to place in any corner. Rebounding not only benefits your physical fitness but also your immune system, lymphatic drainage, and bone strength. Try placing a rebounder in your hallway, so you'll be reminded to do a few bounces every time you walk through your home, or place one in front of your TV.

The Plan

1. Decide what type of exercise you are going to do. (i.e. jumping jacks, burpees, etc.)

2. Decide what time of day you are going to do it. (i.e. when you get home from work)

3. Decide what days of the week you are going to do it. (i.e. every day or every other day)

Action Steps

1. Then, add your new movement routine to your Treatment Schedule. This will help you keep track of it and make sure it gets done!

2. Set an "exercise appointment" on your phone's calendar to remind you to exercise.

3. Track your symptoms on the Symptom Calendar and see how they improve (or worsen) with movement. Remember, if your symptoms get worse, you're exercising too much.

4. Questions? Ask people in the Facebook group (fb.com/groups/fixyourfatigue) questions like these:

   a. *What are your favorite exercises?*

   b. *What's the best way to get exercise in during a busy day?*

   c. *What's the best time of day you like to exercise?*

5. Post videos of yourself working out in the Facebook group!

6. Continue eating more meat and vegetables and avoiding grains and sugars.

7. Congratulations on completing another chapter!

8. In the next chapter, Stacy is going to help you Fix Your Emotional Health!

Chapter 7:
Fix Your Emotional Health

by Stacy Scheel Hirsch, MES, ACC, CDWF

I asked my wife, Stacy, to write this chapter. Stacy had chronic fatigue for three years, and the most powerful treatments she found were ones that helped her to change her emotional landscape and recondition her stress response. Through various practices and therapies, she targeted her brain and her emotions and became aware of the role emotional distress played not only in getting sick but also in sabotaging her healing. Ultimately, she reclaimed her energy and went on to achieve more happiness than at any other time in her life. Now as a lifestyle and personal growth coach, she helps others connect with their wholeness and find their way through chronic illness.

Background

"The number one root of all illness, as we know, is stress." ~
Marianne Williamson

When I became sick with chronic fatigue, I was no stranger to stress, although, at the time, I probably wouldn't have labeled what I was going through as stressful. It felt normal and not that different from how everyone else was living. Mentally, I identified with my life as an adventure or a puzzle to be solved, but the more telling sign was how I was relating emotionally.

In the five years before I became ill, I lived in six different cities in four states, traveled around the world, completed a 150-mile trek in Nepal, started a new business, ran a marathon, trained as a yoga teacher, completed three ten-day silent meditation retreats, went gluten-free, and bought my first home, a 1924 fixer-upper. These were all experiences I chose with great intention and enthusiasm.

If my life had only followed the trajectory I had set, then perhaps I would have never become ill. But that isn't how reality works. Running at equal pace alongside my goals and plans were the relationship missteps; two painful breakups with the same guy, the purchase of a cute San Diego bungalow that fell through when my engagement ended, the rebound relationship that crushed my self-esteem, and the real-life challenges of being self-employed and trying to grow my business while living and working from the construction project I called my home. These perceived setbacks and failures weighed heavily on my mind and heart.

Emotionally, I begin to relate to the adversity I was experiencing with fear, worry, and a sense of failure. On a deeper, unspoken level, I began to doubt my ability to successfully navigate my life, as I focused on all the ways I felt deficient. With each setback, I felt more and more disconnected from the life I wanted to live. My emotions became heavier and more burdensome, and I became more reactionary to the world around me.

Although my emotional suffering was obvious at times, I didn't characterize it as stressful. It was suffering, and we all suffer. I didn't have a complete understanding of what stress was or how the body responds to perceived threats – from the mind or from the environment. I believed if I was determined, I could power through any challenge or setback and override any difficult emotion with sheer will. I wasn't aware that my stress response system was still operating on programming that was wired as far back as the womb. (I will talk more about this when I discuss stress.) As life continued to present more obstacles, my old wiring became more and more active, and my reactions intensified as I began to see threats all around me.

Additionally, I failed to notice how the parts of my life that I labeled as more positive – a new home, a promising career, travel to foreign countries – were also contributing to my overall stress burden. It wasn't the events themselves that were stressful, but how I was relating to them. Worry was the main tool in my toolbox, and although it could be highly motivating, it was also exhausting.

Not understanding the complex interaction between my thoughts, my emotions, and my nervous system left me powerless against the physiologic changes happening underneath the surface. As more fragmentations from childhood became visible, I became more and more dysregulated until I depleted my reserves and entered a chronic state of fatigue, resulting in a complete flat line of my cortisol levels and a myriad of symptoms I had no idea how to fix.

It became clear that my physical body was taking cues from my emotional-mental landscape. Childhood emotions along with thoughts of scarcity and "not being enough" began to show up as physical deficiencies in my body. My cortisol was depleted along with other key nutrients like magnesium, B6, chromium, glutathione, etc., making it difficult for my body to carry out essential functions. As my emotional burden increased, so did the stress on my physical body.

It was a lonely, uncertain time, but I was determined to regain my health and better understand what happened. My symptoms were guideposts if I chose to learn from them, and that is what I did. Healing came in small doses as I accepted my present state of being, nourished my body and mind, and learned new, more powerful, and supportive ways to interact with the world around me.

What is Emotion?

Emotions are central to our human experience. We celebrate and embrace emotions of joy, gratitude, love, and awe while we do our best to avoid the pain of emotions such as anger, jealousy, sadness, and grief. Some people categorize emotions as either positive or negative, yet regardless of the label, each emotion plays an important role in connecting us with our human experience. Emotions are messengers, each speaking their own language.

Karla McLaren in her book, *The Language of Emotions: What your feelings are trying to tell you,* writes, "Emotions alert us to specific trouble, and they do so without any subterfuge. If we're aware enough to listen to them – if our attention is focused and our minds are centered – our emotions will be able to contribute exactly what we need to move into and then out of any trouble imaginable. When we become able to hear and respond to our emotions effectively, we become able to understand the deepest language of our souls. With the support of our fully awakened emotions, those unceasing and abundant energies, we'll be adequate to any situation, any issue, or any trauma."

Emotions are complex reactions worthy of our attention. There is lots of science on this, but let's keep it simple.

The emotional experience has three components.

1. **Subjective experience**: how we experience our emotions.

2. **Physiologic response:** how our physical body responds to our subjective experience.

3. **Behavior or expressive response**: the outward signs of how an emotion is being experienced.

We could also include the belief that cognition or "meaning making" is what connects the stimulus with the emotion. For now, your goal is to understand how your emotional and physical health are delicately intertwined and how optimizing both can help you recover your vitality.

Subjective Experience

How we experience our emotions is completely subjective, meaning it is individualized and unable to be measured. Numerous things influence our subjective experience and shape our perceptions of our emotional world. Some of these include our gene expression, the culture we live in, adversity, poverty, safety, health, family of origin, education, generational trauma, and our physiology.

Anger for one person may be threatening and dangerous, while for another it may be nothing more than frustration. How we experience anger can change from day to day or be mixed with a flood of other emotions.

Physiologic Response

The sympathetic nervous system, which manages the body's fight-or-flight reactions, controls the body's subjective experience of emotion. The amygdala, part of the limbic system in the brain, is made up of two tiny almond-shaped structures that are sensitive to fear and threatening situations. It reacts to our emotions and patterns in our physical environment faster than our conscious awareness can detect. (See the Fix Your Adrenals chapter for more information on the fight-or-flight response.)

Behavior Response

This is the component of emotion most people are familiar with because it is often easy to see. We raise our voices, wave our hands, we begin to sweat, or our face turns red. Why do some people blush with embarrassment while others don't? It is the subjective experience of the emotion that determines the expressive response.

Emotional Regulation

From an evolutionary perspective, and first written about by Charles Darwin, emotions keep us alive. Fear guides us away from danger, while love and desire ensure we procreate.

When we can no longer respond effectively to the ongoing demands of our environment, we become less organized in our thoughts, actions, and interactions. We enter a state of emotional dysregulation. Our responses become exaggerated, we overreact, we take on unappealing behaviors, and we are more likely to create chaos, drama, or conflicts. Emotional dysregulation is often relational and triggered by those closest to us or by those in positions of power.

Symptoms of Emotional Dysregulation

Challenges with our ability to regulate our emotions can manifest in a wide array of symptoms. For me, it began with how I related to common, everyday life stressors. I might raise my voice or sink into despair. It was painful, but it seemed mostly normal. As more dysregulation surfaced, it resulted in difficulty sleeping, depression, night terrors, fatigue, anxiety, and panic attacks.

Symptoms of emotional dysregulation may include:

- Difficulty sleeping, insomnia

- Chronic fatigue, low energy, apathy

- Physical symptoms with no apparent cause

- Anger that is difficult to control

- Difficulty quieting the mind

- Obsessive-compulsive behaviors

- Loss of sexual desire

- Difficulty making decisions

- Brain fog or memory issues

- Difficulty tolerating social activity, the need to avoid others

- Erratic behaviors, easily agitated, mood swings

- Feeling overwhelmed, on the edge, or hopeless

- Racing thoughts

- Engaging in risky behaviors to relieve stress or numb

- Withdrawal or isolation from other people

- Increase in negative or difficult emotions

According to the popular website Mercola.com: *"the American Medical Association (AMA) states 80 percent of all health problems are stress related, and even the conservative Centers for Disease Control and Prevention (CDC) has stated that 85 percent of all diseases appear to have an emotional element."*

What we feel and how we feel matters.

Stress and Emotional Well-Being

"The truth is that there is no actual stress or anxiety in the world; it's your thoughts that create these false beliefs. You can't package stress, touch it, or see it. There are only people engaged in stressful thinking."
~ *Wayne Dyer*

Stress, like emotion, is highly individualized. Your nervous system begins to form while you are still in your mother's womb and continues to wire during the early years of your life. This wiring happens differently for each person, depending on the support available in the environment. Without the proper support, an individual can experience difficulties in self-regulation throughout their lives, leaving them more vulnerable to stressors in their environment. The good news is that you can re-wire.

Most of us are familiar with the concept of stress, but few of us take the time to assess the various stressors in our lives or attempt to understand the underlying emotional triggers and internal conflicts that impact our well-being. Your thoughts, feelings, and experiences form your beliefs. It is these beliefs that are often at the root of stressful moments. How can you become more mindful of this process? How do you shift your subjective experience and create healthier physiologic responses?

What we also know is that moderate amounts of stress and tension can be motivating and provide opportunities for our brains to grow and learn. With enough higher functioning available during a stressful episode, we can examine the thoughts, emotions, and beliefs that are leading to the tension.

The tricky part is knowing when you cross a threshold, where moderate stress starts to become overwhelming and chronic, and where you can no longer regulate your emotional response.

The graphic below depicts a continuum between healthy stress and distress. It shows:

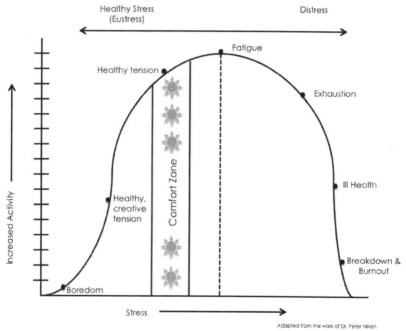

The Human Function Curve

- A low amount of activity combined with too little stress or tension results in boredom.

- When activity increases and one becomes more engaged with life, there is the potential for healthy or creative tension moving a person into a comfort zone. Inside this zone, a person functions well with the proper amount of motivation to feel productive and without the overwhelm that often accompanies greater activity. People often refer to this as a flow state. Our emotional state is easily regulated, and we feel resilient.

- If activity and tension continue to increase, a person may move into a space between comfort and the first signs of fatigue. The early signs of distress may appear as this is where old fragmentation may surface in response to increased tension.

- If we are experienced in the realm of self-care, we may recognize the early signs of distress and take action to avoid more tension, while creating opportunities to reconnect with our comfort zone. This is the space where resilient people engage their support system and avoid crossing the threshold. They read the signs and determine what needs to be addressed.

- When we do not know what to look for, or we don't recognize the early warning signs of distress, we may begin to feel tired with long bouts of fatigue. Exhaustion and other symptoms follow, and if we remain in a state of dysregulation, a breakdown is inevitable, resulting in a chronic state of fatigue and complete burnout.

How do you learn to stay in your comfort zone? Take care of what arises when it arises. Become equipped with the right information and attuned in a moment-to-moment awareness.

It requires you to know yourself, your needs, and your healthy limits and then be equipped to respond accordingly.

This type of awareness is elusive for many people. We often aren't encouraged to know ourselves or to ask for what we need. We get disconnected from our bodies and our emotional selves. We feel pressured by those in our lives and by our high expectations. We search for ways to stay in control, even if it means drifting toward greater distress.

This can also be challenging if you feel the stressors in your life are out of your control, for example, if you experience an infection in your body, long-term illness, a sick loved one, chronic poverty, neighborhood violence, politics, or world events. Understanding what to do doesn't always mean you can make these stressors disappear. When you cannot remove the stressor, you need to look at how you can respond differently or find support to buffer the impact of the stressor. Stress that remains constant changes the brain and impacts the stress response system, creating more stress in the body and increasing the risk of developing chronic health conditions such as fatigue.

Early Causes of Emotional Dysregulation

"Traumatized people chronically feel unsafe inside their bodies: The past is alive in the form of gnawing interior discomfort. Their bodies are constantly bombarded by visceral warning signs, and, in an attempt to control these processes, they often become expert at ignoring their gut feelings and in numbing awareness of what is played out inside. They learn to hide from their selves".
~ Bessel van der Kolk

Adults living with high stress or those with chronic health conditions, such as fatigue, are often unaware that toxic stress experienced as a child, and the adaptations they made to survive their unmet needs, may be partially responsible for their symptoms. Some of my clients believe their chronic fatigue is a byproduct of getting older. They have come to expect the failure of the physical body because it happened to their parents or it happens to everyone with age. It is difficult to grasp that disease processes may have been set in motion as far back as childhood, long before their first symptoms appeared.

Physicians Vincent Felitti and Robert Anda were the first to study the link between childhood adversity and adult health outcomes. In 1995 they surveyed 17,000 Kaiser Permanente patient volunteers about their exposure to ten types of childhood trauma, or Adverse Childhood Experiences (ACEs).

An ACE was defined as a stress-inducing event that was chronic and unpredictable. The ten adverse experiences they chose from the research were:

1. Physical abuse

2. Sexual abuse

3. Emotional abuse

4. Physical neglect

5. Emotional neglect

6. Mother treated violently

7. Household substance abuse

8. Household mental illness

9. Parental separation or divorce

10. Incarcerated household member

That survey data was compared with a patient health history for each participant. The results showed that adverse childhood experiences were much more common than anyone had previously thought, with two-thirds of individuals reporting at least one adverse childhood experience. Researchers followed participants over time and determined that ACEs have a dose-response relationship, meaning the more ACEs you have, the greater your risk as an adult for developing chronic health conditions and engaging in risky health behaviors.

There are other adverse childhood experiences that can be equally damaging to a child such as bullying, generational trauma, homelessness, racism, homophobia, illness, accidents, a traumatic birth, chronic hunger, and family financial stress.

What about the adults who live with the consequences of an environment that failed them as a child? What about those with a history of trauma who are now experiencing fatigue and want to get back to living life?

Fortunately, there are tools for people like us! I will be discussing these in the sections on practices and therapies.

It is difficult to find doctors who work with adults, who understand the connection between illness and childhood adversity, and have the tools to treat mysterious and debilitating symptoms. That is what excites me most about this book. Dr. Hirsch has designed an approach to healing fatigue that gets to the root causes of the illness, including emotions. In my opinion – and even traditional medical providers will agree – emotional health is almost always at the root of physical symptoms. Once you have symptoms, there are real physical problems you must address.

In the past ten years, there has been a dramatic increase in research exploring brain science, epigenetics, emotional well-being, and resilience. This data, combined with the functional medicine tools and protocols discussed in this book, provide powerful opportunities to regain your health and re-connect with the person you were always meant to be.

Testing

The ACEs assessment is meant to be used as guidance in assessing one type of risk factor. There are other risk factors that can contribute to ill health such as genetics, diet, and other lifestyle choices.

As your ACE score increases, so does the risk to your physical and emotional health. An ACE score of 4 or more can be significant, increasing the likelihood of chronic pulmonary lung disease by 390 percent; hepatitis, 240 percent; depression 460 percent; and suicide, 1,220 percent.

In one study, exposure to childhood trauma was associated with a 3- to 8-fold increased risk for Chronic Fatigue Syndrome across different trauma types.

Use the Resilience Questionnaire to reflect on the supportive factors that helped you navigate childhood.

The Devereux Adult Resilience Survey can help you reflect on your current strengths and make a plan for how to improve your overall well-being.

You can find these questionnaires in the free member area of our website (fixyourfatigue.org/members).

Your Potential to Heal in Body and Mind

*"When people clear out their trauma, compassion is their natural state.
Compassion is part of our nature,"*
~ Gabor Maté, MD

Resilience is the ability to rebound from emotional distress, trauma, and adversity. It is about having the capacity to respond when your stress response gets activated. It's not about pushing yourself out of your comfort zone and powering through your symptoms. It is much more subtle, and it is grounded in your willingness and ability to listen to your body and emotions and compassionately respond to what surfaces.

What does resilience look like? People who are resilient have a certain level of confidence and understand their strengths and abilities. They can solve problems and are effective at communicating, even when things are challenging. When strong emotions arise, they can manage their feelings without alienating others.

It is never too late to become more resilient, to stop tolerating life and begin to listen to what your symptoms are trying to tell you. The research suggests that there are numerous things you can do to strengthen your ability to respond to life's challenges such as cultivating more social support, practicing mindfulness, staying physically active, nurturing a growth mindset, and reframing painful or challenging emotions. The next section will provide more information on practices and therapies that increase resilience. I have listed a few to get you started, but you can find more at LifeTakesPractice.com.

Practices

Once you understand how your emotional health may be playing a role in your fatigue, you can start using practices and therapies to support your overall healing. I have been working with practices for the past twenty years and using many of the therapies I describe below. You can find a comprehensive list of my foundational practices at LifeTakesPractice.com.

- **Gratitude:** There is an abundance of scientific research demonstrating that practicing gratitude on a regular basis can improve your overall health and sense of well-being. Studies have found that a gratitude practice can help you overcome traumatic events and increases your resilience, strengthens your immune system, lowers blood pressure, and reduces symptoms of illness, so you feel less bothered, supports you in taking better care of our health, improves your sleep and strengthens your relationships.

- **Self-Compassion:** Research shows that people who practice self-compassion cope better with stress than those who are more critical. Self-compassion reduces your tendency to catastrophize negative situations, experience anxiety following a stressor, and avoid challenging tasks for fear of failure. Self-compassion can help you cope when you experience negative life events.

Kristin Neff, Ph.D., a researcher and author, has identified three elements of self-compassion:

- *Self-kindness*: being kind to yourself in times of suffering. Recognizing that failure and disappointment are a part of life and using self-kindness to moderate your emotional response to stressful or challenging moments.

- *Common humanity*: recognizing that we all suffer and that setbacks and difficulties happen to everyone.

- *Mindfulness*: taking a balanced approach to your emotional state. Holding your negative thoughts and emotions with mindful awareness and avoiding becoming overly reactive.

- **Writing:** Dr. James W. Pennebaker has conducted much of the research on the health benefits of expressive writing. It is believed that the act of thinking about a traumatic or stressful event while also tuning into and expressing the emotions helps people process the experience and understand the greater meaning. It provides a structure for managing the anxious thinking and helps bring more organization to a person's system.

- **Meditation:** Many believe that meditation is one of the most effective ways to moderate stress and increase our emotional intelligence. The practice of meditation helps people cultivate a state of mindful awareness. This state can help neutralize stressful thoughts and emotions by bringing us into the present moment's reality. At LifeTakesPractice.com, I have designated meditation as a foundational practice because everything in your life is impacted by the degree to which you are mindful.

Therapies

- **Emotional Freedom Techniques (EFT)** is an energy psychology practice that can be used to manage or reprogram your stress response. EFT works on the same meridians used in acupuncture, but instead of needles, one uses the fingers to stimulate specific energy points on the body. While focusing on a problem, negative emotion or stressor, you tap the energy meridians on your body and verbalize specific positive affirmations. This process changes the emotional circuitry of the body and removes energetic blocks. The technique is simple and easy for anyone to learn and begin practicing immediately. Search for a practitioner at eftuniverse.com and thetappingsolution.com.

- **HeartMath** is a scientifically proven stress management system that uses tools and technology to connect the head with the heart, much like the practice of meditation. Communication between the heart and brain influences perception, emotional processing, and higher cognitive functions. Research has demonstrated that intentionally focusing on positive emotions can create more physiologic harmony within the body, shifting your relationship away from stressful thoughts, emotions, or traumatic experiences. Learn more at heartmath.org.

- **NARM (NeuroAffective Relational Model)** is a somatic psychotherapy that focuses on supporting an individual in restoring vital connections in three key areas of life experience: physiological, psychological, and relational. The NARM framework is built on exploring five biologically based core needs that are essential to healthy development.

These include our needs for:

1. *Connection*: the capacity to be in touch with your body and your emotions and to be in connection with others.

2. *Attunement*: the capacity to attune to your needs and emotions and to recognize and reach for physical and emotional nourishment.

3. *Trust*: the capacity for healthy dependence and interdependence

4. *Autonomy*: the capacity to set appropriate boundaries, say no, set limits, and speak up without guilt or fear.

5. *Love-sexuality*: the capacity to live with an open heart and to integrate a loving relationship with a vital sexuality.

When these biological needs are met, you are better able to develop core capacities that support you in becoming a healthy and vibrant adult. When a biologically based core need is not met as a child, or only partially met, predictable emotional and physical symptoms result: a decreased capacity for self-regulation, a diminished sense of self, and compromised self-esteem. By paying attention to your emotions, you can begin to let go of those survival patterns you needed as a child but that no longer serve you as an adult. With this awareness, you can now establish a better way of relating to yourself and the world around you. You can find a practitioner at drlaurenceheller.com/practitioners.html.

- **Eye Movement Desensitization and Reprocessing (EMDR)** is a research-supported technique used in psychotherapy to alleviate the stress associated with painful memories, adverse life experiences, and post-traumatic stress. You can find a practitioner at emdr.com. GoodTherapy.org maintains a searchable database of therapists that have verified credentials, offering another way to find an EMDR practitioner in your vicinity.

- **Hakomi** is a mindfulness-centered somatic psychotherapy. At its core, it is designed to create a safe space for people to become more aware of their present moment experience. Transformation happens when emotions and the physical body are integrated. This allows for a reorganization of core beliefs. As your system becomes more organized and coherent, you feel a greater range in your mental, physical, and emotional states. You can find a practitioner at hakomiinstitute.com.

- **Neurofeedback** helps a person train themselves to directly affect brain function. Sensors are placed on specific areas of the head corresponding to different parts of the brain. The brain is then provided feedback, training the brain toward greater regulation. There is promising clinical evidence that Neurofeedback helps to reset the brain's stress response point and improve cognitive functioning and energy levels.

- **Flower essences** are believed to work on a subtle level, through the electrical system of the body, like the meridian system in acupuncture. They help balance negative emotional states, making room for the positive emotions to surface. You can find flower essences online or in health food stores.

- **TRE (Trauma Release Exercises)** offers exercises to release deep muscular patterns of stress, tension, and trauma. Most of the evidence for the effectiveness of TRE is anecdotal at this time. Find a practitioner at traumaprevention.com/.

- **Dynamic Neural Retraining System** is a neuroplasticity-based treatment to stop the flood of stress hormones that lead to increased inflammation in the body, poor detoxification, and immune function and sensory perception issues. Learn more at retrainingthebrain.com/.

Summary

In this chapter, we learned about the distinct components of emotion and how emotion interacts with our physiology to engage our stress response system. We highlighted the signs of emotional distress and how to recognize when we have moved from our comfort zone toward greater distress. We also looked at hidden stressors in the form of toxic childhood stress and how some chronic health issues can sometimes result from the dysregulation that began as a child. Finally, we reviewed several practices and therapies that have been found helpful in reregulating our nervous system, reshaping our brains, and supporting the path back to wholeness.

The Plan

1. Start a practice of gratitude. Every day, write down three things you are grateful for in your life.

2. Consider incorporating other practices into your life like self-compassion, writing, and meditation. You can learn more about the practices I mentioned in this chapter and other practices at LifeTakesPractice.com.

3. Watch this video on Emotional Freedom Technique (EFT) and start practicing it throughout the day whenever you feel stress or anxiety. https://youtu.be/pAclBdj20ZU

4. Research the list of therapies to learn more about how you may incorporate them into your healing protocol. Search for practitioners in your region. You may also want to determine which practitioners work by phone or online if you cannot find a qualified practitioner in your area.

5. Get support! Find a coach, therapist, or someone who is dedicated to supporting you along the way. It can be a challenge to stay on track and still see the big picture, particularly when your internal form of resilience has been "powering through" or ignoring your body. You may need regular support until you can begin to build a new form of resilience in your system and through your behaviors and practices.

Action Steps

1. Download the Practice Planner worksheet from the member area and begin to build your practice plan.

2. Start a practice. You decide which one. I recommend starting with gratitude. Take small steps and begin implementing.

3. Set alarms on your phone to remind you when to practice. Sticky note reminders can help too.

4. Visit LifeTakesPractice.com to learn more about the art of practice.

5. Contact practitioners of the therapies that resonate most with you. Before calling, make a list of questions you would like to ask. Here are some examples:

    a. *What licenses or certifications do you have?*

  b. *How long have you been practicing?*

  c. *What experience do you have working through some of the issues I am experiencing?*

  d. *What is your ideal client?*

6. Download the ACEs and Resilience Questionnaires from the member area at fixyourfatigue.org/members.

7. Questions? Ask people in the Facebook group questions like these:

  a. *Which of these therapies have you used with success?*

  b. *What time of day do you like to do your practices?*

  c. *What have you noticed from doing your practices?*

  d. *How has working on your emotional health affected your fatigue?*

8. Continue to implement the lifestyle changes you have made and the previous treatments.

9. Congratulations on completing another chapter! I know these therapies and practices can change your life the same way they have changed mine!

10. Next, Dr. Hirsch brings together all of the lifestyle habits we have been discussing and shares how he incorporates them into his life!

Chapter 8:
Fix Your Day for Success

For most of my life, I have struggled with prioritizing my health. I always had something else that was more important to do. Where did it get me? I had fatigue and was forced to prioritize my health and create systems to keep me healthy. I found that if it wasn't on my calendar, it didn't get done. I started scheduling everything in my life.

My Life

People who are successful in life create habits and routines that allow them to reach their goals. If you want to be successful, model yourself after someone who has achieved what you want. This is what I try to do in my life. The following is the compilation of the habits that I do in my life based on what have learned from others.

Here is my daily regimen that includes my food, water, movement, supplements, and emotional practices. Please note, this is what my ideal day looks like, but I'm far from perfect.

See which habits you can apply to your life.

- I wake up at 6 a.m. and drink 20 ounces of water with a pinch of sea salt. I have a whole-house water filter (Aquasana.com), so all the water in my house is filtered.

- I meditate for thirty minutes using the Holosync® system. I think about situations that have been challenging for me and uncomfortable emotions, and I process these and practice Emotional Freedom Techniques (EFT/tapping) to help resolve them. I practice breath-walking, incantations, gratitude, and visioning to start my day off right (per Tony Robbins).

- Sometimes I meditate in the sauna. I write down any notes from my meditation session.

- I move my body depending on my energy level. I may do some jumping jacks or gentle yoga stretches to get my day going.

- I take a shower (in filtered water) using fragrance-free, non-toxic (Alaffia) African Black Soap for my body and hair.

- I eat a breakfast that consists of a protein (like bacon, turkey bacon, sausage, and/or eggs) and a vegetable (like steamed or sautéed kale with onions and/or cabbage). I also like to eat a nut and fruit cereal (occasionally with gluten-free granola) that I mix up in the mornings. It consists of soaked and dehydrated walnuts, pecans, and fresh apple or banana in coconut milk. I chew each bite until it is liquid to maximize digestion and provide an easy way to take my supplements.

- I take my supplements with breakfast out of the AM/PM pill organizer that I filled over the weekend.

- I drive my daughter to school, and we listen to musicals on the way. After I drop her off, I make work and personal phone calls or listen to podcasts and courses on topics in medicine on my way to my office.

- When I get to the office, I drink another 20 ounces of water. I have an Aquasana countertop water filter at the office.

- I have a mid-morning snack around 10 a.m. of nuts, seeds, or meat bars like EPIC or Tanka Bites. I take an adrenal support supplement during this time.

- I drink another 20 ounces of water with a pinch of sea salt fifteen to thirty minutes before lunch. I take adrenal and mitochondrial support supplements at this time.

- For lunch around 12 p.m., I eat leftovers from dinner the night before (usually meat with vegetables) or a fresh salad with lots of vegetables and organic lunch meat. We prepare our lunches on Sunday for the week. Frequently, I go for a ten-minute walk after lunch with some of our staff or do jumping jacks.

- For an afternoon snack around 3 p.m., I eat nuts, seeds, or meat bars like EPIC or Tanka Bites. I take adrenal support at this time if needed.

- When I get home from work around 5 p.m., depending on my energy level, I will do ten burpees or jumping jacks. As your energy gets better, you can work up to a seven-minute workout with interval training.

- For dinner around 5:30 or 6 p.m., we eat organic, grass-fed, free-range meats (beef, lamb, chicken or turkey) with organic vegetables (peas, string beans, broccoli, cauliflower, carrots, kale, chard, collards, etc.). We cook it all together like a stir-fry (but use coconut oil, not soy sauce) or cook the meat separately and cook the vegetables in a steamer basket. We use sea salt and olive oil on our food after it has cooked. I take some of my evening supplements at this time.

- After dinner, we listen to music (dance party!), clean-up, connect with each other, and I read with my daughter. I take my evening anti-microbial (bug killing) supplements at this time.

- I then work on the business (my goal is to eventually work only on relaxing, creative tasks), spend time with my wife, Stacy, and occasionally watch some TV. I keep lights low and blue light blockers on my computer and phone to allow my body to get ready for sleep.

- I drink another 20 ounces of water with a pinch of sea salt one hour before sleep (at 8:30 or 9 p.m.).

- I start getting ready for bed at 9:30 p.m. I do some push-ups, sit-ups, and stretches before bed. I am in bed at 9:45 or 10 p.m. and read a pleasure book for fifteen to twenty minutes. I take my activated charcoal supplement. Lights out at 10 or 10:30 p.m.

Which habits do you want to apply to your life?

My goal is to have the following elements in my life every day:

1. **Mindfulness**: A mindfulness practice like meditation. Holosync® is audio tracks that help you meditate and evolve emotionally.

2. **Food**: Healthy food that is organic, grass-fed, paleo, and low-allergy. Regular snacks to keep my blood sugar stable.

3. **Water**: Water consumption on a regular basis away from meals. I add sea salt occasionally to support my adrenal glands.

4. **Music**: I try to sing and dance as often as possible.

5. **Education**: I want to keep growing and learning for my mental, emotional, and professional health, so I listen to people who have achieved what I want and emulate them.

6. **Movement**: I have several times during the day when I move my body.

7. **Sleep**: Sleep is prioritized with a 10 p.m. bedtime and good sleep habits.

8. **Connection**: I connect with my community at my daughter's school, my work family, and my home family.

What elements do you want in your life?

The Plan

1. Take the time now to schedule your ideal day. If you could structure it any way you wanted, what would it look like? Dream the dream.

2. When you write it down, it comes to fruition. So go ahead. Put down this book, pull out a piece of paper and start writing. I'll wait....

Action Steps

1. Use the Practice Planner (from the member area) to determine which practices and habits you want to implement

2. Now, add your new schedule from your ideal day to your phone's calendar to remind you what to do and

when. When the reminder goes off, stop everything and complete the task.

3. Get some accountability. Share with the Facebook group:

   a. *How your energy has been affected by going to sleep at 10 p.m.*

   b. *Goals that you'd like help sticking to*

   c. *What your goals are for your life*

4. Continue to implement the lifestyle changes you have made thus far.

5. Congratulations on completing another chapter!

6. Get excited for Step II: Replace deficiencies!

Step II:
Replace Deficiencies

Chapter 9:
Fix Your Adrenals

I woke up after eight hours of sleep, and I felt awful. The fatigue was heavy on my back and my eyelids. After hitting the snooze button a few times, I buried my face into my pillow and pushed myself back into child's pose. "Okay, time to get up, let's do this, you can do this," I thought as I tried to motivate myself to action. I got out of bed and immediately became light-headed. I knew that by the time I got to work, I'd be a bit better, but only until three o'clock when my energy crashed, and I had to push through the brain fog and the fatigue once more. My adrenal glands were not happy.

Background

The adrenal gland is a little triangular organ about the size of a walnut. There are two, and they sit atop each of your kidneys. The central part of the adrenal gland, the adrenal medulla, is the part that produces epinephrine (adrenaline) and norepinephrine, two primary acute stress hormones. The outer part of the gland, the adrenal cortex, produces the stress hormone cortisol, sex hormones, and aldosterone, which helps control blood pressure and salt balance. I will be focusing on cortisol since its dysfunction leads to adrenal fatigue. Adrenal fatigue is a primary cause of chronic fatigue.

The stress hormones epinephrine, norepinephrine, and cortisol allow you to react quickly in dangerous situations by fighting or running away. This phenomenon is commonly known as the fight-or-flight response.

Historically, this stress response was needed for a short amount of time: when you encountered a wild animal, an enemy or during times of famine. Unfortunately, in today's society, we are inundated with daily stressors that cause a chronic, continuous release of these stress hormones. This, in turn, leads to chronic stress and dysfunction.

Cortisol has many functions in the body. It provides the energy we need to get out of bed in the morning and function during the day. It regulates the immune system, insulin, blood sugars, inflammation, tissue repair, electrolyte (salt) balance, circadian rhythm, thyroid, and sex hormone function. There is a reason many practitioners consider the adrenal gland the "sentinel gland"—it's the conductor of the symphony that is the body and an important regulator for many other glands and systems.

Prolonged physical, mental, energetic, or emotional stress can deplete your cortisol and lead to adrenal fatigue, a syndrome that depletes the hormones produced by the adrenal gland.

Symptoms

You may have adrenal fatigue if you have some of following symptoms:

- Difficulty being out of bed for more than a few hours a day because of fatigue

- Feeling tired regardless of the length of time one sleeps

- Feeling unusually tired in the morning and the afternoon around 3 p.m. Do you need a cup of coffee to get moving in the morning?

- Low blood pressure (top number less than 110)

- Orthostatic hypotension (dizziness or lightheadedness when moving from sitting or lying to a standing position)

- Cravings for sweets/sugar and/or salt (potato chips!)

- Sleep problems (hard time falling asleep and/or staying asleep)

- Lack of interest in sex

- Poor memory or "brain fog"

- Increased inflammation (and pain)

- Weight gain, especially around the middle

- You get every cold and flu bug going around

- A feeling of overwhelm for tasks that you used to be able to handle easily

- An improvement in your symptoms when on vacation

- A second wind if you stay up after 10 p.m.

- Post-exertion malaise (fatigue after exerting oneself). An individual with adrenal fatigue may exercise (or even just wash the dishes!) for ten or fifteen minutes, and then have to sleep the rest of the day.

As I mentioned in the first chapter, in 2015, the United States Institute of Medicine renamed CFS as systemic exertion intolerance disease (SEID). The three symptoms they say must be present for diagnosis are impaired day-to-day functioning because of fatigue, malaise after exertion (physical, cognitive, or emotional), and unrefreshing sleep. The symptoms must also be accompanied by either cognitive impairment or orthostatic intolerance (low blood pressure), or both.

Sound familiar? Essentially, they are describing adrenal fatigue.

The Causes of Your Adrenal Fatigue

Lots of practitioners talk about adrenal fatigue as THE cause of your chronic fatigue, but unfortunately, they don't ask the next question:

What are the causes of your adrenal fatigue?

Adrenal fatigue can develop gradually over time, or it can come on more acutely, typically following an illness or an infection, or after a particularly stressful period in your life. Normally, when you experience a stressful event, the adrenal glands produce more cortisol to regulate it and keep the homeostasis (balance) present in the body. I have found that most of my patients with adrenal fatigue experience one or more major stressors (physical, mental, emotional, or energetic) before developing symptoms of adrenal fatigue. These stressors require the adrenal glands to produce more and more cortisol in response to the stressor until the adrenal glands can no longer keep up with the demand and become "burned out."

Physical stressors may include motor vehicle accidents, surgeries, too much exercise, or toxicity from what I call the *usual suspects*: heavy metals, chemicals, molds, infections, emotions, electromagnetic frequencies (EMFs), and allergies.

Mental and emotional stressors include relationship stress, breakups, divorces, the death of a loved one, work stress, past emotional trauma, abuse, and adverse childhood events.

Energetic stressors include batteries, electricity, and EMFs that disrupt our DNA (genetic material) and damage our cells. Not spending enough time in nature will also disrupt the body's energy fields.

When taking a patient's history, I listen to the story of their health since birth, paying close attention to the presence of any of these stressors. The more stressors (or "hits") over time, the more strain has been placed on the adrenal gland and the more likely they will have adrenal fatigue and its consequences.

It's estimated that up to 80 percent of adults experience adrenal fatigue during their lifetimes, yet it remains one of the most under-diagnosed illnesses in the United States. Conventional medicine does not yet recognize adrenal fatigue as a distinct syndrome.

Symptoms vs. Testing

So, based on the symptoms above, do you think you have adrenal fatigue? Symptoms are the most important criteria we look at when diagnosing, but as human beings, we like data. We want to see the chemistry inside our bodies and a documentation of dysfunction. I like to test, and patients like to test, but for some causes, testing may not be as important. This is the case with adrenal fatigue. If you have most of the symptoms listed previously, you probably have adrenal fatigue. However, the more complex a patient's case, the more testing is needed to discern symptoms that cross over into other causes. For example, the 3 p.m. energy crash is typically caused by a drop in cortisol; however, sometimes it is due to a drop in T3, one of the thyroid hormones. This interplay between the thyroid, adrenals, and sex hormones is quite intricate, and this is where testing is vital.

Testing

So, how do we test for adrenal dysfunction? I look mainly at blood values, but I have used saliva and urine testing as well. They are all good options and are reliable under the evaluation of an experienced clinician.

It is important to remember that all of this is *data collecting*. Your symptoms, your labs, your history, your exam, and your treatment successes and failures are ALL important and necessary. My wife, Stacy, says, "Failure is merely data collection," and she is right. You need all of this information to determine what next steps to take on your healing journey.

It is also important to remember that all labs are imperfect. Yes, you read that right; all of them. Lab values are a snapshot in time that measures a biomarker located in the area at that particular moment. So, take them with a grain of salt and use all of the data mentioned above to come to a conclusion. When I lecture to physicians, I tell them, "If you lean too heavily on your lab results, you will fall over."

I prefer blood testing for the sake of cost and convenience. Blood testing requires a fasting blood draw in the morning. Saliva testing involves spitting into little tubes four to five times over the course of a day, which is measured and compared with the normal cortisol curve (below). Cortisol should be high in the morning and then gradually fall throughout the day, allowing you to fall asleep easily at night. The graph below shows normal cortisol levels throughout the day.

We always want to remind ourselves what "ideal" or "optimal" looks like so we know where we are heading and what we want to achieve.

The middle line shows us a normal picture of cortisol throughout the day. It starts high and decreases over the course of the day.

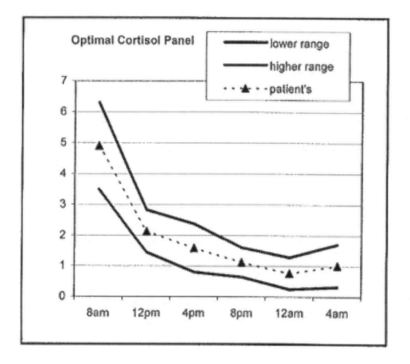

In addition to cortisol, it's important also to assess levels of DHEA (the hormone dehydroepiandrosterone), which you can think of as the adrenal reserves. DHEA is an anti-aging hormone with whole books written about it. It compensates for abnormal cortisol levels.

What Tests do I Recommend?

For blood testing, I recommend that you test:

- Morning cortisol level (between 7 and 9 a.m. ideally). The serum (blood) cortisol normal range is between 15-25 (not "free cortisol").

- DHEA-S. The "S" on the end of the DHEA is a sulfate group that lasts longer in blood and is a better measurement of active DHEA. The normal range is 150-200 for women and 300-400 for men.

You can find these tests at FYF.MyMedLab.com, DirectLabs.com, PrivateMDLabs.com, or HealthLabs.com.

For saliva testing, you can use the Hormone Saliva – ZRT test (at FYF.MyMedLab.com). It also includes sex hormones, which is a better deal. Use the lab's reference ranges.

Tip: If your thyroid function is low, your cortisol and DHEA will be falsely elevated trying to compensate for the low thyroid. For example, if you have three symptoms of adrenal fatigue, a cortisol level of 16 (normal range), and your thyroid function is low, you have adrenal fatigue *even though* your cortisol level is in the normal range. This is because, in reality, the cortisol level is probably less than 15, but it has increased itself to compensate for low thyroid function.

Stages of Adrenal Fatigue

The progression of adrenal fatigue can be broken down into seven stages, with stage 7 being the most severe. With each progressive stage, every organ and system in the body are more profoundly affected. Stages 6 and 7 (adrenal exhaustion) involve nearly complete adrenal failure. Most people with adrenal fatigue seek treatment when they are somewhere between stage 2 and stage 5. Those in stages 6 and 7 produce virtually no cortisol. If you want to see what these curves look like, visit StopTheThyroidMadness.com.

The Seven Stages of Adrenal Fatigue

- **Stage 1**: Cortisol levels begin to rise, but DHEA compensates; body still balanced so no obvious symptoms

- **Stage 2**: Cortisol continues to rise, but DHEA is unable to compensate; body cannot keep up with stress; mild symptoms warn "trouble ahead"

- **Stage 3**: High cortisol, low DHEA; anxiety and even "panic attacks"; this state uniquely marked by anxiety and exhaustion combined; insomnia common

- **Stage 4**: Cortisol levels drop, DHEA remains low as body's hormone reserves have been exhausted; difficulty going to sleep and waking in the morning because cortisol levels are higher at night

- **Stage 5**: Cortisol continues to drop, but DHEA rises temporarily because body no longer attempts to adapt; extreme weakness and fatigue, possibly bedridden

- **Stage 6**: DHEA levels *above normal* in body's last gasp to protect itself before giving up completely; ACTH does not function, so cortisol does not respond; rare to see individuals in this stage

- **Stage 7**: Complete adrenal failure; cortisol flat-lines

My approach to treating adrenal fatigue, as with most conditions, is to *start low and go slow*. We can always ramp up the therapy, but a gentle approach allows the body to accommodate and incorporate the physiological responses to treatment gradually. The illness did not develop overnight, and I've learned that patients respond best to a gradual healing process of baby steps. And I like results, so I'm going to be recommending treatments that work.

My goals are to:

1. Replace the cortisol deficiency so that the person can function at their best every day.

2. Heal the adrenal glands with vitamins and minerals.

3. Reset the relationship between the brain and the adrenal glands.

4. Decrease excessive cortisol release (from a chronic fight-or-flight or startle response)

5. Remove the causes

Treating with Supplements

Some of my favorite supplement interventions for adrenal fatigue are:

- DHEA

- Eleuthero root

- Adrenal Stress End

- Licorice root

- Adrenal cortical extract

- Tyrosine

- Vitamin B2

- Vitamin B5

- Chromium

- Hydrocortisone/cortisol (Cortef)

I am going to discuss each of these and then summarize my recommendations at the end of the chapter.

The amino acid tyrosine stimulates the medulla (and the thyroid), and vitamins B2 and B5 are very restorative to the adrenal gland. Licorice root allows the cortisol produced by the adrenal cortex to last longer by inhibiting its conversion into cortisone. I have found adrenal cortical extract also to be quite helpful for those who are more sensitive to supplements.

For those individuals who feel "wired and tired," Cortisol Manager by Integrative Therapeutics contains phosphatidylserine, theanine, and other calming herbs that allow you to keep your edge while decreasing your anxiety and "fight-or-flight" reactivity.

Adaptogens

Adaptogenic herbs are excellent at helping the body adapt to stress. These special herbs are grown in "stressful environments." Adaptogens support better brain-gland communication, which becomes impaired under adrenal fatigue. In other words, these herbs improve the signals between the brain and endocrine glands, which include the thyroid, adrenals, and ovaries or testes. If you are tired, adaptogenic herbs will increase your energy. If you are anxious and stimulated, these herbs will produce a calming effect.

Adaptogenic herbs include:

- Ashwagandha

- Asian ginseng

- Astragalus

- Eleuthero root

- Rhodiola

- Holy basil

My favorite adrenal support is eleuthero root, and it is found in a product called Adrenal Px by Restorative Formulations. I have been very impressed with its ability to improve energy and balance hormones.

If you react strongly and only need a small dose of supplements and medications for the desired effect, I recommend starting on adrenal cortex extract alone or chromium. When we're born, we have fourteen times more chromium in our adrenals than we have in the rest of our body!

Adrenal agents last for only about three hours in the body, so take them in divided doses throughout the day. I recommend taking them in the morning, at noon, and at 3 p.m. They do not need to be taken on an empty stomach. The 3 p.m. dose is optional, depending on your energy demands later in the day. Don't take any supplements after 4 p.m., because they can be stimulating enough to interfere with your sleep.

If these treatments are not producing the results you desire, then work with your practitioner to increase the dosages.

Sleep tip: It's important to remember that by fixing your adrenal fatigue that your sleep problems will improve. This is because your sleep issues are most likely a circadian rhythm problem. Your circadian rhythm is your body's natural sleep-wake cycle. When you are tired during the day, your body thinks you are supposed to be awake at night.

By taking adrenal supplements in the early part of the day, you are recreating the natural rhythm, and it will become easier to fall asleep and stay asleep during the night.

Advanced Adrenal Recommendations

IMPORTANT! *I only recommend high doses of licorice root when working with a healthcare provider. While it is generally safe, it can have many dangerous side effects that need to be monitored. These include high blood pressure, low potassium, swelling, and heart palpitations.*

If more energy is needed and cortisol remains low (less than 15 in blood on serum cortisol), I bring out the biggest gun: prescription Cortef (hydrocortisone). Your healthcare provider must prescribe this. Due to inaccurate, conflicting, or outdated information, some physicians believe prescribing cortisol for adrenal fatigue is not safe, but I am convinced that it is. It's made the difference for many of my patients. *Safe Uses of Cortisol* by Dr. William Jefferies is an excellent resource. Ask your doctor to read it.

Cortef is a steroid. If you have heard about the side effects associated with prednisone, a common steroid used for autoimmune diseases, you may have concerns about taking it. Let me put your mind at ease. The cortisol your body produces is a steroid as well! Cortef brings your cortisol levels into the normal physiologic range that the adrenal glands would be producing if they were functioning correctly. And Cortef is a much smaller dose than the lowest dose of Prednisone. I am only recommending that you replace what is deficient and not take any more than that.

This brings me to an important point. We always want to mimic nature the best we can. We want to replace deficiencies to a place of optimal functioning, but not beyond it. We want to restore your body to how it was before you became unwell.

Treat the Causes and Reduce the Stressors

Treating the physical symptoms is only the first step. Once you start to feel better, it's important to begin addressing the causes of the problem: the sources of stress that compromised your adrenals in the first place.

Stress, as we discussed, can have physical, mental, emotional, and energetic (spiritual) elements.

The physical stress from heavy metal toxicity, infections, chemicals, molds, and food allergies must be addressed. I will be discussing each of these in subsequent chapters.

Mental and emotional stressors are just as important. Here is a list of action items, but don't get overwhelmed. See Stacy's Fix Your Emotional Health chapter for more information. Besides restoring your adrenals, choose one thing to do from this list:

- **Make a plan**: this can help to manage the stress that arises from juggling relationships, family, finances, and work. If you're uncomfortable enough with your situation, then you know it's time to make a significant change. This may be changing who you spend time with, a change in hours, or even a change in your job.

- **Go to bed at 10 p.m.** This will help reset your circadian rhythm, and you'll avoid missing your sleep window. Lights go off at 10, so start getting ready before then. I'll have more tips for you in the sleep chapter.

- **Start a gratitude practice**: You will experience a noticeable reduction in your level of stress. Every day say out loud or write down three things you are grateful for. You can learn more about the research and how to start a gratitude practice here: LifeTakesPractice.com/gratitude

- **Start a stress-reducing technique**: you have probably neglected yourself in the midst of feeling overwhelmed. Effective stress management tools include meditation, mindfulness training, yoga, tai chi, and Emotional Freedom Techniques (EFT or tapping)—and there are certainly many others. Pick one and go for it! Start slow, maybe once a week, and increase as your energy grows. I have found Holosync® to be incredibly helpful for me. It is an audio recording of music that puts your mind into a meditative state.

- **Start having more "YOU" time!** You are worth it! You deserve thirty to sixty minutes of "YOU" time each day to take care of yourself. Tony Robbins calls this your "hour of power." You cannot serve others from an empty well. You need to fill your well up with gratitude, calm, peace, nourishing food, and exercise before you can go out into the world and help others. It has made a big difference in my life and the lives of my patients. Put the time on your calendar and make it happen. You will be amazed at how *you* can transform your life!

Other lifestyle action items (some of which we discussed in Step I already) include:

- Avoid caffeine in chocolate and coffee. Unfortunately, coffee whips the adrenal glands, making them less functional, and requires you to drink more coffee to get through your day. Caffeine also can stay in your body for up to twenty hours, so your morning cup may be affecting your sleep!

- Drink more water and sea salt. When your adrenals aren't working, you're not making enough aldosterone to keep the salt in your body. So, you need to start putting sea salt on your food and in your water. Start with a pinch of sea salt per glass of water and increase slowly. If it tastes too salty, you've put in too much! Consume three to four liters of water per day in between meals. Try it and see what a difference it makes!

- Eat protein and fat every two hours and stop eating grains and sugar. When you eat grains and sugar, your blood sugar will spike and your insulin reacts to push it into your cells. Cortisol is then released to manage the insulin. When your blood sugar is stable, your cortisol can be preserved for other adrenal functions. Good sources of fats are nuts, olive oil, coconut oil, and avocado. I like Epic meat bars for protein and fat as a snack between meals. Your ideal diet will be meat and vegetables. A quarter of your plate at every meal should be meat and the rest vegetables (one-quarter can be starchy vegetables). A plate of varied, colorful vegetables is ideal.

- Add exercise and movement as you are able. Exercise is a powerful tool for mitigating stress, but only if you have enough energy to tolerate it. I usually don't recommend exercise for the first few months of treatment unless your energy levels are good and you don't feel worse after exercise. Start low and go slow. Too much exercise will deplete the adrenals. I recommend you start exercising when your energy level is at a 6 out of 10 or higher and that you start slow. I recommend five to ten jumping jacks or burpees per day as a starting point.

Consider if you may be "spiritually (or energetically) stressed." When ill or in intensive treatment, a person is operating in "survival mode." The end of treatment marks an important crossroads. Once you feel better, you will have the energy to begin thinking about your life's purpose:

- Are you doing what you want to be doing in this world?

- Are you living your passion or purpose?

- Do you feel fulfilled?

- Have you been in "survival mode" with only enough energy to put one foot in front of the other each day?

- When you have enough energy what will you do with it?

- How will your life be different?

I encourage you to visit <u>LifeTakesPractice.com</u> for tools and support in pursuing a richer life. As you know, my wife, Stacy, suffered from chronic fatigue for three years. An important part of resolving her fatigue involved exploring opportunities for mental, spiritual, and emotional growth. She now experiences a greater level of energy and a stronger sense of well being than she has ever felt in her life. She took her personal experience and her experience with her clients and created <u>LifeTakesPractice.com</u> to help you change your life for the better.

Take the next step to who you want to be.

Summary

Adrenal fatigue is a syndrome that develops when your adrenal glands are no longer able to meet the demands of intense or prolonged stress. The primary symptom is fatigue not alleviated by sleep, although symptoms can be quite diverse, as the entire body tries to compensate when the adrenal glands are unable to keep up.

Nearly 80 percent of adults may experience adrenal fatigue at some point during their lifetimes, and yet conventional medicine does not recognize it as a distinct syndrome.

Adrenal fatigue can develop gradually over time or come on acutely after a significant physical or psychological stress. It progresses through seven stages, depending on the severity of adrenal depletion. Common symptoms include morning fatigue, afternoon energy crashes, low blood pressure, cravings, insomnia, and increased inflammation.

Laboratory testing for adrenal fatigue can be done using saliva, blood, or urine. Two primary assessments are cortisol levels and DHEA, and how those levels fluctuate over the course of a typical day.

Treating adrenal fatigue involves replacing function and removing the causes. Stress management and lifestyle changes are necessary if recovery is to be permanent.

Working with a medical professional, preferably a provider trained in functional medicine, is always advised for treating the nuances of your condition. This type of practitioner can assist you with laboratory testing and interpretation of the results, as well as customize your treatments and monitor your progress to make sure you're proceeding safely,

The Plan

For those patients who have adrenal fatigue based on their signs, symptoms, and laboratory testing, here's what I recommend.

I always recommend that you start only one new thing every four days to be able to observe any reactions you may have.

1. Start Adrenal Stress End: 1 cap in the morning and noon. Not after 4 p.m. Take with food. Watch for side effects of the licorice root in this product: feeling wired, insomnia, high blood pressure, heart palpitations or swelling. If this occurs, stop the product and start BioAdreno 1 cap in the morning, noon, and at 3 p.m. Increase to 3 caps three times per day as able. If BioAdreno is too stimulating, take chromium picolinate 1000 mcg 1 to 6 caps/day. It's a great treatment for sensitive folks, just not very strong.

   Note: 3 p.m. doses are not needed if you do not have an energy crash between your last dose and 10 p.m.

2. Start Adrenal Px: 1 cap in the morning, at noon, and at 3 p.m. Increase in one week by 1 cap per dose. Max

4 caps three times per day to get cortisol levels into the normal range. Decrease if you experience any agitation, insomnia, or feeling wired (rare).

3. Start DHEA 25 mg per day (for men) and increase up to a max of 75 mg/day as needed to fix your blood levels. For women, start at 5 mg per day and increase up to a max of 25 mg per day.

4. Start Cortisol Manager: 1 tab two times per day if you are feeling overwhelmed, anxious, or have insomnia. It can also be helpful if you are feeling "wired and tired," if you startle easily, and for high cortisol readings.

I recommend taking the above supplements until energy increases to a 7/10 and symptoms and laboratory values improve into the normal range. Once the causes of the adrenal fatigue are remedied, you can wean down as able.

Action Steps

1. Order the new supplements discussed in this chapter and start the ramp-up! You can find them under the Adrenal Support category in our online store here: us.fullscript.com/welcome/drhirsch

2. Add your new supplements to your Treatment Schedule & Calendar (free in the member area)

3. Set alarms on your phone to remind you to take your supplements

4. Track your symptoms on your Symptom Calendar (free in the member area)

5. Questions? Ask people in the Facebook group (fb.com/groups/fixyourfatigue) questions like these:

    a. *Which adrenal support product do you like the best?*

    b. *How long did it take you to ramp up on your Adrenal Px before you got to the right dose?*

    c. *What adrenal support products have you tried and which ones have worked for you?*

6. Continue to implement the lifestyle changes you have made.

7. Congratulations on completing another chapter!

8. Get ready to Fix Your Thyroid in the next chapter!

Chapter 10:
Fix Your Thyroid

I had beautiful curly hair down to my shoulders when I entered residency in 2004. But by the end of residency three years later, my hair was dry and brittle. My hands and feet were cold and swollen. I had brain fog, memory loss, and constipation. I had hypothyroidism.

Background

Thyroid disease is one of the most common health problems we face today. The majority of people with thyroid dysfunction have hypothyroidism. Hypothyroidism ("hypo-" means low) is a condition where the amount of thyroid hormone in your body is less than what is needed for optimal function.

According to the American Thyroid Association, more than 12 percent of the US population will develop a thyroid condition during their lifetimes, and more than half will be unaware that they have a problem. Women are five to eight times as likely as men to develop thyroid problems.

The thyroid gland is shaped like a butterfly and found directly below the Adam's apple, covering the throat. The thyroid produces thyroid hormones (mainly T3 and T4) that regulate the body's metabolism and affect numerous vital body functions including breathing, heart rate, body temperature, and energy level. When your thyroid hormone levels are optimal, every system in your body works better.

Hyperthyroidism ("hyper" means high) is a condition characterized by the presence of too much thyroid hormone in the body. It can cause fatigue as well, but it is less common, so we are going to focus on hypothyroidism.

Hypothyroidism is a major cause of chronic fatigue.

Thyroid Physiology (Function)

Optimal thyroid health depends on effective communication between the brain and the thyroid. The hypothalamus (in the brain) stimulates the pituitary gland (also in the brain) to produce TSH, the chemical messenger that is then sent to the thyroid with instructions on how much thyroid to produce. Free T3 and free T4 are the two main hormones produced by your thyroid gland. The "T" represents tyrosine, an amino acid, and the number refers to the number of attached iodine molecules—either three or four. These free hormones send feedback to the brain (the hypothalamus and the pituitary), so thyroid levels can be regulated. For example, during hypothyroidism, the level of thyroid hormone in the body is low. The body sends a message to the brain that it needs more thyroid hormone. The brain sends TSH to the thyroid with a message to make more thyroid, and the thyroid complies.

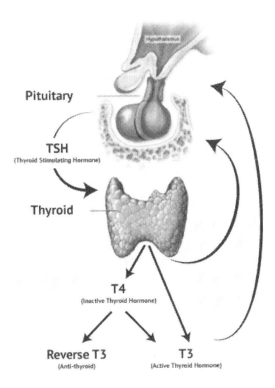

The body converts T4 into T3 at the cellular level and in the liver using iodine, selenium, and iron. Although T4 is referred to as the "inactive" thyroid hormone, this is a bit of a misnomer because T4 is not inactive—it has important functions and in many cases needs to be replaced. We'll discuss this more when we get to thyroid replacement.

During times of stress, T4 will be converted to reverse T3 instead of T3, and the person will experience symptoms of low thyroid.

Interestingly, new research also shows that our mitochondria (the energy centers of every cell in the body except red blood cells) act on cells to increase their absorption of thyroid hormone. This absorption can be compromised if toxins damage the mitochondria.

Autoimmune Hypothyroidism

Hashimoto's thyroiditis (or autoimmune hypothyroidism) is the most common cause of hypothyroidism, accounting for approximately ninety percent of cases.

Iodine and selenium deficiencies can also cause hypothyroidism, but this is less common in first world countries.

Hashimoto's is an autoimmune disorder in which the immune system attacks and breaks off parts of the thyroid gland, resulting in suboptimal thyroid hormone levels. Thyroid antibodies are indicators of autoimmune thyroid disease.

Unfortunately, the natural progression of autoimmune hypothyroidism is a continuous destruction of the thyroid gland, and thyroid levels decrease over time. When a piece of thyroid tissue breaks off, thyroid hormone is released from the cells, and people may report symptoms of hyperthyroidism for a short time. These symptoms include tremors, heart palpitations, insomnia, headaches, weight loss, agitation, anxiety, diarrhea, bulging eyes, and sometimes a goiter (enlargement of the thyroid gland). Then, symptoms of hypothyroidism worsen as the thyroid hormone is cleared and they're left with lower levels of thyroid hormone than they had before.

Consequently, Hashimoto's is two conditions that need to be treated: an autoimmune disease and a deficiency in thyroid hormone levels.

Another autoimmune condition that affects the thyroid is Graves' disease. This occurs when the immune system stimulates the thyroid gland to *overproduce* the thyroid hormones. The immune system produces antibodies that mimic the TSH (normally coming from the pituitary gland).

These TSH antibodies then stimulate the thyroid to produce too much of the thyroid hormones, and hyperthyroid symptoms result.

Symptoms

You may have hypothyroidism if you have some of the following signs and symptoms:

- Chronic fatigue

- Cold extremities (hands and feet)

- Memory loss

- Hair loss

- Lower leg swelling

- Constipation

- Dry skin and hair

- Brittle nails

- Weight gain or difficulty losing weight

- Elevated blood sugar or diabetes

- Elevated cholesterol

- Elevated blood pressure

- Depression, anxiety

- Heart palpitations or arrhythmias

- Poor cognition ("brain fog")

Undiagnosed thyroid disease can increase your risk for other serious conditions, such as cardiovascular (heart and blood vessel) disease, Alzheimer's disease, osteoporosis, and infertility.

It has been exciting to observe how improved thyroid function influences other laboratory markers. Cholesterol levels, inflammatory markers, cardiovascular risk markers, congestive heart failure (heart strain) markers, blood sugar, and diabetes markers *all* improve when thyroid hormone is optimized.

Testing

I want your body to be strong before you address the causes of the autoimmunity, so I support it with thyroid supplementation and medications. I do this based on symptoms and lab testing. Here are my optimal ranges for these lab values:

- TSH: 0.5 - 1.5 ulU/ml

- Free T3: 3.0 – 4.0 pg/ml

- Free T4: 1.2 – 2.0 ng/dl

- Reverse T3: less than 24 ng/dl (optional)

- Anti-thyroglobulin antibody: less than 115 IU/ml

- Anti-thyroid peroxidase antibody: less than 34 IU/ml

These levels are only a guide and should be considered data to complement your subjective experience (your symptoms). If your labs show adequate hormone levels, but you are still having symptoms of low thyroid, ask your doctor to trust your experience and increase your thyroid dose. *Note: if your adrenal hormone (cortisol) is low, treat this first before raising your thyroid dose.*

Conventional medicine relies very heavily on the TSH which is, unfortunately, quite inaccurate once someone is on thyroid medication. Free T3 and free T4 are the free (bioavailable) fractions of these hormones and far more reliable as markers of thyroid function. Dr. Datis Kharrazian, DC, does a great job of explaining this in his book *Why Do I Still Have Thyroid Symptoms?*

T4 converts to reverse T3 instead of T3 during times of stress from any of the *usual suspects*. The result is lower T3 levels and low thyroid symptoms, including fatigue.

Tip: It's also important to note that free T4 and free T3 thyroid levels may be falsely elevated if cortisol (the main adrenal hormone) is low. This is because the thyroid is compensating for low adrenal function. Once cortisol is in the normal range, you will get a lower (and more accurate) reading of your thyroid hormones.

Elevated thyroglobulin and thyroid peroxidase antibodies confirm a Hashimoto's diagnosis. However, values will be variable based on cortisol levels, stress, immune system function and the time of day the sample is drawn. Since autoimmune thyroid is ninety percent of all hypothyroidism, we can usually assume the cause is autoimmune, and antibody testing is less important. Tracking the antibodies can be helpful, though, to determine the success of treatment.

Once the causes of the autoimmunity are being treated, antibody levels should improve. If they do not, you need to look for other causes.

Do You Have Hypothyroidism?

At this point, you should have your labs back, and you can evaluate if you have a thyroid problem.

You probably have hypothyroidism if you have the following:

- A TSH greater than 1.5

- Free T4 less than 1.2

- Free T3 less than 3

- Signs and symptoms of low thyroid

You probably have Hashimoto's (autoimmune) disease if any of your antibodies are elevated and if you have hypothyroidism and you don't live in Michigan. (Keep reading; I'll explain!)

The Causes of Autoimmune Thyroid Disease

Why is autoimmune thyroid disease on the rise? It can largely be attributed to today's highly polluted world. Once again, it's the *usual suspects*!

1. Heavy metals such as lead, mercury, aluminum, and cadmium

2. Toxic chemicals such as herbicides, pesticides, formaldehyde, fluoride, bromine, and plastics made with toxic chemicals such as BPA

3. Electromagnetic frequencies

4. Mold and mycotoxin (mold toxins) exposure

5. Allergies; usually food allergies such as gluten, dairy, soy, corn, and others

6. Infections, such as Epstein-Barr virus, cytomegalovirus (CMV), *Bartonella*, Lyme disease, Yersinia, H. pylori, and Mycoplasma

7. Your emotions and beliefs affect your health. Many people believe there is a like between disliking oneself and autoimmune diseases.

These toxins trigger the immune system in several ways. First, they damage cells, releasing the components of the cell into the bloodstream. Cellular components aren't supposed to be seen in the blood, so the immune system creates antibodies to remove them. These antibodies end up attacking other cells that have the same components. Second, these toxins hide in the cells of the thyroid, and the immune system does its best to remove them but damages the thyroid in the process.

It is important to remember that many of these toxic particles get into your body through the foods you eat, the water you drink, and the air you breathe. This is why it is so important to eat organic food, drink filtered water, and breathe clean (filtered) air that is free of molds, fragrances, and auto exhaust.

The first step in halting the progression of autoimmunity is to remove the causes. I will discuss treatments for these factors triggering autoimmunity more fully in their respective chapters.

Did you know that the most common time for a woman to acquire an autoimmune disease like Hashimoto's disease is after she gives birth? This is because after delivery there is a huge decrease in progesterone. During pregnancy, progesterone is a wonderful anti-inflammatory that prevents the immune system from reacting to any of the *usual suspects*. This is a protective mechanism to make sure the mother's immune system does not attack the fetus. At delivery, when progesterone drops, the immune system awakens and starts producing antibodies to the *usual suspects* that have been left unchecked during pregnancy. This may result in Hashimoto's disease.

The best thing that you can do for your health and to quiet your autoimmunity is to stop eating gluten. Gluten triggers autoimmunity, damages our intestines every time we eat it (whether we have symptoms from eating it or not), and increases inflammation. It should be illegal! I go more into gluten in the chapter on food allergies.

Th1 and Th2 Autoimmunity

Th1 and Th2 refer to two types of immune processes in the body. "Th" refers to T-helper cells, which are lymphocytes (white blood cells) that identify what they believe to be foreign particles in the body that need to be removed, and then produce cytokines (another immune cell) in response. In the case of autoimmunity, these Th cells attack your body's tissues.

- Th1 cells are involved in "cell-mediated immunity" and are the body's first line of defense against these foreign invaders inside the cells. Th1 cells tend to be pro-inflammatory and usually involve organ-specific autoimmune diseases.

- Th2 cells are involved in "humoral-mediated immunity," stimulating antibodies against extracellular invaders (those found in blood and other body fluids). Th2 cells tend not to be inflammatory and usually involve systemic autoimmune disease and other chronic conditions.

If your immune system is functioning properly, both types of T-helper cells work together to keep things in check. But when your immune system goes awry, one type can become overactive and suppress the other, which makes symptoms worse. In most autoimmune conditions, either Th1 or Th2 will be dominant.

Slowing Down Autoimmunity

We need to do everything we can to halt the progression of the autoimmunity and preserve the thyroid gland. We do this by removing the *usual suspects* and by calming down Th1 and Th2 autoimmunity with high dose vitamin D and fish oil, and low dose naltrexone (LDN).

LDN causes the body to release natural opiates (endorphins and enkephalins), which stimulate T-regulatory helper cells to slow down the autoimmune reactivity. This is important because you want to prevent damage to your thyroid and autoimmunity in other parts of your body. Once you have one autoimmune process underway, other autoimmune conditions can develop, like rheumatoid arthritis or lupus.

Natural Treatment for Hypothyroidism

I am a big believer in natural medicine. It can be very powerful and work very well. I prefer to use it as long as the natural treatment is safe and strong. Unfortunately, when treating low thyroid, we usually need both the natural and the prescription treatments. In college, I learned from playing the card game *euchre* not to "send a boy to do a man's job." In medicine, this means using the treatment that you *know* will work. If I *think* a natural treatment will work, but I *know* that a medication will work, I should use the medication as long as there are no significant side effects. This is because I want to make sure you get results right away so that you can get your life back. If we mess around with natural remedies for six months and you do not see any improvement, I'm not helping you to the best of my abilities and knowledge.

Here are the natural treatments that I use:

- Thyroid glandulars

- Iodine (seaweed, kelp)

- Magnesium

- Iron (spinach, beef)

- Selenium (Brazil nuts – 2 per day)

- Adaptogens

The same adaptogenic herbs we use with the adrenals, we can use here as well. These herbs will regulate the relationship between the brain and the thyroid gland. Thyroid glandulars take over some of the function of the thyroid and allow it to rest and repair itself. Vitamins, minerals, and foods provide nutrients to the thyroid to make T4 and T3 and to convert T4 to T3.

Thyroid Px is the product I like to use that has a combination of these natural treatments.

If I need something stronger, I like to use Priority One's Thyroid 65 glandular. If the patient needs more support, I turn to prescription medications.

The Iodine Controversy

Dr. David Brownstein has done a lot of work with iodine and has many success stories using it to reverse Hashimoto's and thyroid disease.

Unfortunately, I tried his protocols a few years ago and did not have success. I did find that some people tolerated iodine well, but some people do worse. I have not seen it resolve Hashimoto's. I have seen it increase antibodies and the size of a thyroid goiter, so please use iodine with caution. If you feel worse on it, or if your labs indicate that the iodine is worsening your condition, please stop taking it.

I believe the disparity in our experiences is because Dr. Brownstein is located in Michigan, where the population is significantly iodine-deficient due to iodine deficiency in the soil and consequently, the food. The soil in Olympia, Washington, where I live and work, is iodine-sufficient, so our population does not have the same problem.

Thyroid Medications

When it comes to choosing thyroid medications, my motto is to go with what works. Some practitioners believe that there is only one type of medication to treat low thyroid. For conventional medicine providers, this is usually levothyroxine (T4). Occasionally I'll see an endocrinologist prescribe liothyronine (T3). Naturopaths and functional medicine providers seem to prefer desiccated thyroid (Armour, WP Thyroid, or Nature-Throid) because it is more natural, coming from animal sources. However, I practice personalized, individualized medicine, and I know that every patient is different, and they require a different combination. For example, patients who are chemically sensitive (have negative reactions to normal dosing of medications, supplements, fragrances, and foods), do better with synthetic medications. Their bodies are already reacting to their own tissues, so any natural thyroid that you use will trigger another reaction. A patient who is taking a maximum dose of desiccated thyroid but still has low thyroid symptoms, including low T4, will need some levothyroxine.

The forms of thyroid support that I use are:

- Levothyroxine (T4)

- Liothyronine (T3)

- Desiccated thyroid (Armour, WP Thyroid, or Nature-Throid)

I will use brand, generic, or compounded prescription (oral and topical) forms of thyroid medications. I will combine any of these together as needed to get a patient feeling better.

I begin treatment when I am convinced (by symptoms and blood testing) that a patient has hypothyroidism. I usually choose desiccated thyroid to start if the patient is deficient in T4 and T3, but mostly in T3. Desiccated thyroid is natural, dehydrated, and powdered tissue from animal sources, usually cows or pigs. My favorite forms are WP Thyroid and Nature-

Throid for their purity (both by RLC Labs). Armour Thyroid is the most common desiccated form found at conventional pharmacies. However, the last few years it has undergone some reformulating, and there is some concern that it has gluten in it. If a patient reacts, I switch them to Nature-Throid or WP Thyroid. Desiccated thyroid is a strong dose of T3 and a light dose of T4. It works well if you need more T3 than T4. Consequently, based on your labs and your symptoms, you may require T4 augmentation later in your treatment. My typical dosing for desiccated thyroid ends up being one or two grains daily. Each grain is 65 milligrams and contains 9 mcg of T3 and 38 mcg of T4. One grain of desiccated thyroid is considered to be approximately 100 micrograms of levothyroxine (synthetic T4).

If a patient requires T4 only, I will prescribe levothyroxine. I recommend taking it first thing in the morning, thirty minutes before breakfast. It lasts eight to twelve hours in the body, so it only needs to be dosed in the morning.

If a patient requires T3 only, I use the synthetic form of T3, liothyronine. Liothyronine typically lasts three to four hours in the body, so I find dosing every three to four hours is best—morning, noon, and 3 p.m. This schedule seems to help prevent the afternoon energy "crash." If the crash persists in spite of dosage adjustments, it may stem from adrenal dysfunction, rather than thyroid.

Choosing the Right Thyroid Medication

Here are some lab testing scenarios to help you determine which thyroid medication is right for you. In all of these situations, TSH is above 2.

Case #1: If you have a free T4 of 0.9 and free T3 of 3.2, what should you do?

Answer: Since free T4 is low and free T3 is normal, choosing a medication with only T4 is recommended. This is levothyroxine.

Case #2: If you have a free T4 of 0.8 and a free T3 of 2.5, what should you do?

Answer: Since both free T4 and free T3 are low, you'll want to use a combination of T4 and T3. This can be in desiccated thyroid or taking T4 and T3 separately. You would ramp up on the T4 first before adding the T3.

Case #3: If you have a free T4 of 1.4 and free T3 of 2.6, what should you do?

Answer: Since T4 is normal and free T3 is low, then you want to take only T3, liothyronine.

Treating Thyroid Subjectively

Typically, the process to be prescribed thyroid medication is as follows:

1. The patient sees their provider.

2. The provider orders lab tests.

3. They go over the results, and the provider prescribes thyroid.

4. Lab tests are repeated every six to eight weeks to determine the thyroid status. From the time you start taking a dose of thyroid, there is a six- to eight-week delay before results can be measured.

5. This process continues until the right dose is reached, and the patient's symptoms are resolved (if they need only levothyroxine). This may take up to six months.

6. Every six to twelve months the patient will feel worse, so they will return to the provider, who will repeat the process and probably increase the thyroid medication as the thyroid destruction continues.

You can shortcut this process by following my Thyroid Ramp-Up, in which you gradually increase the treatment based on your experience. I typically start my patients on (for example) a dose of WP Thyroid 32.5 milligrams (a half a grain) in the morning on an empty stomach and increase the dose by 32.5 mg every two weeks as long as they are improving and not having any symptoms of hyperthyroidism (too much thyroid). When they experience any of these symptoms (tremors, heart palpitations, diarrhea, anxiety, agitation, headaches, or insomnia), I have them back down to their previous dose. If the patient does not have the awareness to identify these symptoms when they occur, then this treatment is not for them. Your provider may want to see you every two to three weeks to make sure you are on track and not missing any signs of too much thyroid.

Now, if you are going to be subjectively assessing the success of your supplementation, you must recognize when you begin to approach a hyperthyroid state and back off on the dosage to an acceptable level. There is a danger of remaining in a hyperthyroid state: it can cause osteoporosis and cardiovascular problems. When the first hyperthyroid symptoms begin to appear, you must immediately lower your dose back to the previous dose you were taking before the symptoms appeared.

For patients who require only T4 and no T3, I will prescribe levothyroxine. I start them at 25 mcg per day in the morning on an empty stomach and recommend that they increase by 25 mcg every two weeks up to 100 mcg or until they get symptoms of too much thyroid. I only ramp up one medication at a time. Since T4 converts to T3, I will ramp up T4 before T3 to see how much of the T4 is converting to the T3. Otherwise, the patient may become hyperthyroid before reaching the T4 dose they require.

The Nuances to Dosing Thyroid Medications

Thyroid should always be taken on an empty stomach thirty to sixty minutes before breakfast. This is more important for T4 than T3. I will be referring to levothyroxine as T4 and liothyronine as T3. T4 will last for eight to twelve hours in the body. T3 will last for three hours. So, dosing will be different. T4 should be taken in the morning, and T3 should be taken every three hours starting in the morning and ending before 4 p.m. (usually morning, noon, and 3 p.m., like adrenal support) to avoid any insomnia from taking it too late in the day.

The ratio of the T3 to T4 is also very important. Sometimes a patient will have symptoms of low thyroid even though their thyroid labs are in the optimal range. This means that something else is affecting the thyroid's function. It may be an adrenal or sex hormone deficiency or that the T3:T4 ratio is not ideal. To adjust the T3:T4 ratio, you may need to decrease/increase T3 or T4. In this case, desiccated thyroid is not the best treatment. Since the T3:T4 ratio is standardized, you cannot change it for each patient. In this case, I would adjust the ratio by adding or subtracting T3 or T4, depending on the lab results and the patient's symptoms.

It is also important to note that in some cases, synthetics are less reactive for the immune system. I've seen autoimmunity worsen on desiccated thyroids and improve on synthetics.

Please be aware that most of the pharmaceuticals have fillers and/or gluten. This probably accounts for some of the difference between brand and generic medications and why some patients feel better on the brand. Gluten is best avoided because it's a major trigger of autoimmunity. Some pharmacists offer gluten-free products, which I utilize whenever possible.

I want to emphasize the importance of partnering with a healthcare provider who will work with you to resolve your thyroid issues. This may require some assertiveness on your part. Your doctor needs to honor your subjective experience in gauging your response to treatment, rather than "treating a lab report." If your labs look great, but your symptoms continue, I want you to ask your doctor to increase the dose, increasing it by a small increment every two weeks. If the doctor is worried about making you hyperthyroid (and the side effects that come with this), assure them that you will let them know when you experience those symptoms. Your body will let you know when you've taken too much.

When implemented correctly, I have seen wonderful responses to thyroid replacement—increased energy, cessation of hair loss, improved sleep, reduced inflammation, improved blood sugar regulation, and better cardiovascular risk profile. But occasionally, thyroid replacement can make one feel worse, which is usually a sign that the adrenals need attention. There is a beautiful dance that happens between the adrenals, thyroid, and sex hormones; when they *work together,* you will feel good. If you replace one of the "dancers" but are not getting the desired response, you may need to address the other components.

For example, hair loss is usually a symptom of low thyroid. However, I have treated hair loss successfully by boosting adrenal and sex hormone function when they have been deficient. You do not have to live with hair loss!

Thyroid and Heart Health

One of the reasons why optimizing your thyroid function is so important (besides improving your fatigue!) is that it has an amazing effect on many parts of your body. The most dramatic results I have seen have been on the cardiovascular system. Here is a list of how proper thyroid function decreases your risk of having a heart attack or stroke:

- It lowers blood pressure

- It lowers cholesterol and other lipoproteins

- It lowers blood sugars

- It improves congestive heart failure by decreasing the strain on your heart muscle

- It decreases inflammation around your heart and blood vessels

- It decreases the thickness of your blood

So, get your thyroid optimized!

Reversing Thyroid Disease

One of the things that I enjoy most is getting people off of their prescription medications. Medications are very helpful, but they are just a Band-Aid. When you heal the cause, you no longer need them. I have helped people get off of their medications for rheumatoid arthritis, high cholesterol, and high blood pressure (to name a few). I have only recently figured out how to reverse thyroid disease and get people off their thyroid medication!

I have found two ways of doing this. The first way is by treating *Bartonella*, a bacterium that infects the thyroid. I figured this out by chance, and there's a great story that goes along with it in the Infections chapter.

The second way is using Pulsed Electromagnetic Fields (PEMF). I prefer the PEMF by BEMER to improve circulation and absorption of nutrients and oxygen.

I find that when using these therapies, patients who are on thyroid medications become hyperthyroid! When that happens, the patient decreases their thyroid medication by a small amount (e.g. a half grain) every time they have hyperthyroid symptoms until they have completely weaned off it. I find that 80 percent of my patients will wean off of their thyroid medicine completely in three to six months. If they are not able to do this, other causes are getting in the way.

Summary

Hypothyroidism is a significant cause of fatigue today, particularly among women. In addition to fatigue, low thyroid can produce symptoms such as weight gain or difficulty losing weight, hair loss, cold extremities, elevated blood sugar, and poor cognition ("brain fog"). Undiagnosed thyroid issues can increase your risk for other serious health problems, including cardiovascular disease, osteoporosis, and infertility.

Thyroid dysfunction is diagnosed based on a combination of laboratory testing and the patient's subjective symptoms.

Thyroid problems are frequently missed by conventional blood panels, which focus on TSH.

A large proportion of today's thyroid problems are autoimmune, a result of chemicals, heavy metals, infections, and other agents in the environment that are toxic to the thyroid. Hashimoto's disease is the most common cause of low thyroid.

In addition to addressing the causes of the thyroid problem, I use supplementation and medications to support thyroid function. I use desiccated thyroid, levothyroxine (T4), liothyronine (T3), or a combination of these. I start my patients out on a low dose, providing instructions about increasing the dosage, and then I follow up with regular appointments and laboratory monitoring.

The Plan

If you have Hashimoto's disease and you want to slow down your autoimmunity by treating the Th1/Th2 autoimmune imbalance, start the following:

1. Start low dose naltrexone (LDN) 1.5 mg/night and increase by 1.5 mg every week up to 4.5 mg/night. This is a compounded prescription from your medical provider.

2. Start Vitamin D Supreme 20,000 IU/day (4 caps)

3. Start OmegAvail TG1000 (omega-3-fatty acids) 6000 mg per day (6 caps) of combined EPA+DHA

4. I would also recommend resetting the relationship between the immune system and the cause by finding a practitioner who uses low dose antigen and low dose immunotherapy (LDA and LDI).

If you have the signs, symptoms, and labs showing low thyroid, start the following:

1. Start Thyroid Px 1 capsule in the morning. In one week, if you do not see symptom resolution, increase to 2 capsules in the morning. In another week, if you do not see symptom resolution, then add in Priority One Thyroid 65mg below.

2. Start Priority One Thyroid 65mg (thyroid glandular) 1 capsule thirty minutes prior to breakfast on an empty stomach and increase by 1 capsule every two weeks until you get symptoms of hyperthyroidism (tremors, heart palpitations, insomnia, diarrhea, agitation, anxiety, and headaches), then back down by 1 capsule to the previous dose. Recheck labs every six to eight weeks. If you still have low thyroid symptoms once you have reached this dose, you will need to switch or augment with a prescription.

3. Make sure you have supported the adrenals before the thyroid.

If you have ramped up to the maximum dose (hyperthyroid symptoms) on the Priority One Thyroid 65mg and you are still having some of your symptoms of low thyroid, then find a provider to prescribe the appropriate thyroid medication. You will mostly likely need some additional T4 (levothyroxine). See the section on Choosing the Right Thyroid Medication in this chapter.

Action Steps

1. Order the new supplements discussed in this chapter and start the ramp-up! You can find them under the Thyroid Support category in our online store here: us.fullscript.com/welcome/drhirsch

2. Add your new supplements to your Treatment Schedule

3. Track your symptoms on the Symptom Calendar

4. Set alarms on your phone to remind you to take your supplements

5. Questions? Ask people in the Facebook group (fb.com/groups/fixyourfatigue) questions like these:

    a. *Who has good gluten-free recipes? (To avoid triggering your autoimmunity!)*

    b. *How long did it take you to ramp up on your thyroid before you got to the right dose?*

    c. *What thyroid medications have you tried, and which ones have worked for you?*

6. Continue to implement the lifestyle changes you made in Step I and the treatments since then.

7. Congratulations on completing another chapter!

8. Get ready to Fix Your Sex Hormones in the next chapter!

Chapter 11:
Fix Your Sex Hormones

Sarah did not have fatigue. At least she didn't until she hit menopause and stopped sleeping. When I saw her in my office, she had fatigue, a hard time falling asleep and staying asleep, low sex drive, vaginal dryness, hair loss, dry and brittle hair, anxiety, memory loss, agitation, depression, and difficulty making decisions. She wanted her old life back.

Background

The primary sex hormones are estrogen, progesterone, and testosterone. Men and women have all of these, just in different amounts and ratios. Estrogen and progesterone are found in greater amounts in women. Testosterone is the predominant sex hormone in men. They are called "sex hormones" because they regulate the reproductive (sex-related) functions of the body. These include the menstrual cycle and the production of eggs by the ovaries and sperm by the testes.

When men and women have chronic fatigue caused by an imbalance in their sex hormones, it is usually from different hormones. For men, it is usually due to a testosterone deficiency. For women, it is usually due to estrogen and/or progesterone imbalances.

These imbalances can occur at any age but tend to get worse as people get older. The most dramatic shifts in sex hormones occur at puberty, after delivering children (for women), around menopause (for women), and in andropause (for men). Menopause and andropause typically occur around fifty years of age and are characterized by a cessation of reproductive activity and, consequently, a decrease in

164

reproductive (sex) hormone production. I will focus on menopause and andropause in this chapter.

Sex Hormone Excess

Deficiencies are the main imbalance associated with sex hormones; however, there are also cases of sex hormone excess. This is typically from a buildup of estrogen – commonly referred to as *estrogen dominance*. Estrogen dominance symptoms typically occur one to two weeks before menses. It is at this time that the amount of progesterone in the body is supposed to be greater than the amount of estrogen. However, because of the way estrogen is removed from the body and the presence of estrogen mimickers (see xenoestrogens below), estrogen levels may increase, upsetting the estrogen: progesterone balance and causing symptoms of premenstrual syndrome.

Symptoms

Symptoms of imbalances in the sex hormones can be categorized best as deficiencies or excesses.

Symptoms of Estrogen Deficiency

These symptoms are typically found in peri- (approaching menopause) and post-menopausal (after menopause) women:

- Hot flashes

- Vaginal dryness

- Pain with intercourse

- Hair loss

- Memory loss

- Recurrent bladder infections

- Depression

- Joint stiffness

- Light or absent menses

- Weight gain

- Fatigue

- Problems staying asleep

- Increased risk for heart attack and Alzheimer's disease

Symptoms of Estrogen Excess

These symptoms are typically found in menstruating women the week before their menses (periods):

- Premenstrual and menstrual symptoms (bloating, headaches/migraines, abdominal cramping, etc.)

- Irregular periods

- Breast swelling and tenderness

- Fatigue

Symptoms of Progesterone Deficiency

These symptoms are typically found in peri- and post-menopausal women.

- Hard time falling asleep

- Premenstrual symptoms

- Depression

- Anxiety

- Headaches

- Migraines

Symptoms of Testosterone Deficiency

These symptoms are typically found in men and women after fifty years of age or younger when the *usual suspects* are present:

- Decreased libido

- Erectile dysfunction

- Hard time building muscles

- Poor decision-making ability

- Diminished physical performance

- Lack of endurance/stamina

- Depression

- Anxiety

- Increased risk for heart attack, diabetes, and Alzheimer's disease

- High cholesterol

Symptoms of Testosterone Excess

These symptoms are typically found in women with polycystic ovarian syndrome and men on testosterone therapy.

- Anger

- Aggression

- Ovarian cyst growth

- Facial hair growth

- Infertility

- Increased risk for heart attack or stroke (because of blood clotting)

Hormone Imbalance

How many people are walking around with their sex hormones off kilter? Quite a few—perhaps even the majority. One estimate is that nearly 80 percent of women suffer from a hormone imbalance.

The American College of Obstetricians and Gynecologists estimates more than 85 percent of women of childbearing age have at least one pre-menstrual stress symptom as part of their monthly cycle. Most have fairly mild symptoms, but three to eight percent have a more severe form called premenstrual dysphoric disorder (PMDD). Between five and ten percent of women suffer from PCOS, which typically results from elevated androgens. Androgens (like testosterone) may be considered "male hormones," but both men's and women's bodies produce androgens. Androgens have more than two hundred actions in women, including the conversion into estrogens.

The issue of testosterone deficiency in men has become increasingly popular in the media. You may have noticed increasingly frequent advertisements about low testosterone or "low T." In men, testosterone deficiency can produce symptoms such as erectile dysfunction, low libido, osteoporosis, diminished physical performance, and mood and sleep disturbances. It's estimated that more than thirteen million men may have low testosterone, affecting 40 percent of men age forty-five and older. According to one survey, 70 percent of men with low testosterone levels report erectile dysfunction and 63 percent report diminished libido. Low testosterone in men has been associated with an increased risk of mortality (death) from all causes; unfortunately, 90 percent of men with testosterone deficiency never receive treatment.

These statistics point to just how prevalent sex hormone imbalances have become today. The good news is that when managed correctly, modulating and supporting sex hormones can greatly improve your health and quality of life, making your menopause or andropause transitions much smoother.

Testing

The methods I use to assess sex hormone status include patient symptoms and blood, urine, and saliva testing. Blood testing is the most convenient, however, it is only good for assessing testosterone unless the levels of estrogen or progesterone are very high or low. Urine testing is best if you are already receiving hormone therapy, whereas urine or saliva both work well for those not yet receiving hormone therapy.

The urine test that I recommend for post-menopausal women on hormone therapy is the DUTCH Complete-Precision Analytical Inc. Kit (through DirectLabs.com).

The salivary test that I recommend for men and women not on hormone therapy is the ZRT lab Hormone Saliva Test (through FYF.MyMedLab.com).

Here are the blood tests that I recommend for men and women on or off testosterone and their ideal ranges:

Sex Hormone Binding Globulin (SHBG)	20-130 (women), 10-80 (men)
Total testosterone	12-82 ng/dl (women), 500-700 ng/dl (men)
Free testosterone	1.0-2.0 ng/dl (women), 8-15 ng/dl (men)

When SHBG is elevated, it indicates that testosterone levels are low. This is another way of assessing testosterone deficiency.

The Dance of the Hormones

A beautiful dance takes place between the thyroid, the adrenals, and the gonads (ovaries/testes). These glands compensate for each other during times of stress and imbalance. Ideally, when the gonads stop producing sex hormones (as in menopause and andropause), the adrenals and the thyroid should compensate by increasing the production of their own hormones. Sex hormone production is also continued by the adrenal glands. However, in today's high-stress and toxic world, the adrenal gland's function may already be compromised and may be unable to compensate adequately. This results in the hormonal deficiency symptoms of menopause and andropause. Consequently, if adrenal and thyroid function is optimal, an individual will have fewer symptoms of menopause.

Fat Cells Produce Estrogen

Did you know that fat cells produce estrogen? Consequently, the more fat cells a woman has, the higher her estrogen levels will be. This is why women with lower body fat tend to have more challenges with menopause and osteoporosis (which is also dependent on estrogen levels).

Endocrine Disrupting Chemicals

Besides normal life transitions, chemicals in our environment can also disrupt our hormones. One group of chemicals that is particularly disruptive is xenoestrogens (pronounced "zee-no estrogens").

The endocrine system in the human body is made up of glands that produce hormones. These hormones then travel through the body and act on distant sites. Endocrine-disrupting chemicals disrupt hormones by mimicking or interfering with normal hormone function. Also called xenoestrogens, these chemicals can cause symptoms of estrogen excess like painful menses, premenstrual syndrome (PMS), and other menstrual irregularities.

Endocrine disruptors are everywhere—in plastics, packaging materials, foods, medications, personal care products, household cleaners, agricultural products, office supplies, building supplies, cosmetics, fragrances, sunscreens, flame retardants, and more. Unfortunately, no label will say, "contains endocrine disruptors." If you drink beverages from plastic water bottles or apply lotions from plastic bottles made with these chemicals, you may have unusual estrogenic processes taking place in your body.

Xenoestrogens may be driving rates of chronic disease through the roof. In 2012, a comprehensive joint study by the World Health Organization and UNEP concluded we might be significantly underestimating the disease risk from them, including diabetes, obesity, cancer, and infertility. There is abundant evidence that these chemicals are causing our children to reach puberty at increasingly earlier ages. These health risks are exactly why we need to remove these chemicals from our bodies. I will discuss how we do this in subsequent chapters.

The Environmental Working Group lists the top endocrine disrupting chemicals as the following:

- Bisphenol A (BPA)

- Dioxin

- Atrazine

- Phthalates

- Perchlorate

- Fire retardants

- Lead

- Arsenic

- Mercury

- Perfluorinated chemicals (PFCs)

- Organophosphate pesticides

- Glycol Ethers

Now that we know the symptoms of sex hormone deficiencies and why they may occur, let's take a look at how we treat these issues.

Natural Treatment

The symptoms of menopause are no joke. They are incredibly uncomfortable and can change the quality of someone's life significantly. When a woman presents to me in my office with menopausal symptoms, she usually is pretty desperate for relief. I use natural and pharmaceutical therapies to reach this end.

Maca is an adaptogenic herb that can boost sex hormone function by stimulating endocrine glands. Sometimes called "Peruvian Ginseng," maca is a South American adaptogenic root tuber that, when grown under certain conditions, can nourish the hypothalamus-pituitary-adrenal axis (HPA axis). In doing so, it supports the body's production of estrogen, progesterone, and testosterone. I have had success with the product FemmenessencePro by Natural Health International for this purpose. It has its own ramp-up that I will discuss under *The Plan* section at the end of the chapter. In clinical trials, 84 percent of post-menopausal women using FemmenessencePRO experienced a highly statistically significant reduction in menopausal symptoms within two days to eight weeks, with an average of three weeks to experience improvment.

Another herb that can be helpful is black cohosh. Black cohosh can boost estrogen levels and reduce hot flashes. Other therapies that can be helpful include exercising, soy, optimizing adrenal and thyroid hormone function, and consuming an anti-inflammatory Paleo diet of vegetables, lean meat, and no grains.

These herbal and lifestyle remedies can be very helpful. If they do not resolve your symptoms though, I recommend moving on to bio-identical hormone replacement therapy.

Bio-Identical Hormone Replacement Therapy

Bio-identical hormone replacement therapy (BHRT) refers to the use of hormones that are identical on a molecular level to those hormones that we naturally produce in our bodies. BHRT is usually referring to sex hormones, but desiccated thyroid is a perfect example of bio-identical hormones as well.

My mantra in hormone replacement therapy is "start low, go slow, mimic nature, and measure, measure, measure." I learned this from Jonathan V. Wright, MD, who wrote the first BHRT prescription in the United States in the 1980s.

Besides resolving annoying symptoms, optimizing sex hormones has other health benefits, such as reducing the risk of cardiovascular disease, heart attack, stroke, and Alzheimer's disease.

First, Do No Harm

Before we dive into treating with BHRT, let's discuss the safety concerns.

In July 2002, the Women's Health Initiative (WHI) canceled their study and informed all women on HRT (hormone replacement therapy) to discontinue treatment because of the increased risk of stroke, heart attack, breast cancer, and blood clots. Let's take a look at why they may have had these results.

1. **The hormones used were not bio-identical.** Prempro (an oral combination of Premarin and Provera) was the prescription used in the WHI study. Its components are concerning. Premarin is a large dose of horse estrogens. It comes from pregnant mare's urine (hence the name pre-mar-in). Even though horses are from nature, their estrogens are very different from humans.

2. **The dosing was too high.** The estrogens in Premarin are one thousand times stronger than the estrogens made in human bodies. Provera is a large dose of synthetic progesterone that has been shown to increase heart attacks in women.

3. **Oral estrogens were used.** Oral estrogens are processed by the liver and changed into different chemicals. They then essentially become xenoestrogens and can cause cancer and other problems.

4. **Laboratory testing wasn't done**. Conventional medical providers don't check estrogen hormone levels during treatment. They do it for thyroid hormone; why not estrogen? To be sure any treatment is safe requires testing the levels in the body.

Though HRT increases the risk of stroke, heart attack, breast cancer, and blood clots, it is very different from BHRT.

I believe that BHRT can be done safely when the following criteria are met:

1. Only the lowest amount of hormone is used to achieve the desired symptom relief. I tell patients, "we're taking your hormones back to before your symptoms began – a year or two ago, not twenty years ago."

2. Annual urine testing is done to look at hormone levels and the cancer risk ratios (2/16 ratio)

3. Annual ultrasound of the uterine lining is done

4. BHRT is applied topically, not orally (to avoid going through the liver)

5. BHRT is only used for as long as it is needed.

6. Always use more estriol (anti-cancer) than estradiol (more active with a potential to cause cancer)

7. Always use progesterone when prescribing estrogens to decrease the cancer risk

8. Consider using natural anti-coagulants (blood thinners) like fish oils, vitamin E, nattokinase, and serrapeptase

That said, there is *always* a risk when introducing hormones into the body. This is why I have my patients sign a consent form. I want them to know that there are risks, even when using natural, bio-identical hormones. I tell patients that, "the risk we are assuming is the same risk your body had before you went into menopause." If you started having symptoms at fifty years old, but were fine at forty-nine, increasing your hormones to that level is our goal. If you had an estrogen-sensitive tumor growing when you were forty-nine years old, the risk from your own estrogen is the same as the risk from the BHRT. But is it a risk you want to take? Like many things in medicine, you need to assess the benefits and the risks.

The reasons not to prescribe BHRT:

1. History of female cancer (uterine or breast) in the patient

2. History of female cancer in an immediate family member (mother, daughter, sister)

3. History of or genetic predisposition to blood clots (Factor V Leiden, Prothrombin)

4. If the urine test or ultrasound cannot be done

Estrogen Therapy

There are three naturally occurring estrogens in the body: estrone, estradiol, and estriol. For bio-identical estrogen therapy, I recommend a combination of estradiol and estriol (called Bi-est) compounded into a cream and applied to the vulva (outside the vagina) at bedtime. We chose this location because we want to mimic nature by releasing the hormones near the gonads and because the blood vessels and mucus membranes quickly absorb it. In men, this is going to be the anus, because it is the closest mucous membrane to the testes.

The combination of estradiol and estriol supports the benefits of the treatment while decreasing the risks associated with it. Estradiol is great at reducing estrogen deficiency symptoms, but it may promote the risk of heart disease and cancer. To balance this, estriol protects the heart and prevents cancer, but is weakly estrogenic and not great for treating low estrogen symptoms on its own. Consequently, they make a great team. I use more estriol than estradiol in the Bi-est cream to decrease the risks of therapy. I typically use a ratio of 80 percent estriol to 20 percent estradiol. I recommend starting with 0.25 to 0.5 mg of cream, applying 0.2 ml to the vulva each night. If your symptoms of estrogen deficiency are not relieved, increase the dose by 0.1 ml per week until you experience breast tenderness (a sign of too much estrogen), then back down to your previous dose. I call this the Estrogen Ramp-Up protocol. Once you have figured out the right dose for you, check your levels in urine.

I also recommend using progesterone with the Bi-est to provide additional anti-cancer and heart-protective effects. You can add progesterone even without symptoms of low progesterone. I recommend 20 mg added to the cream after you have completed the Estrogen Ramp-Up and you've figured out the right dose of Bi-est for you.

If you don't have access to a medical provider, consider the supplement Ostaderm-V, a fermented plant derived estriol cream derived from wild yam. You ramp-up by 1/8 tsp every week.

Progesterone Therapy

Progesterone can be applied topically as a cream or swallowed as a pill. What?! But what about the risks, Dr. Evan? Didn't you just say that when hormones are consumed orally that they are changed by the liver and can cause cancer? Yes, I did. However, progesterone is *fat* soluble, not water soluble, so it does not get processed by the liver and does not have any of the associated risks. With progesterone, I prefer the oral form because it is more effective in treating insomnia and anxiety symptoms, the two most common progesterone-related complaints that I hear.

To find out the right dose of progesterone for you, use my Progesterone Ramp-Up protocol. Start with one 25 mg capsule of compounded progesterone at night. Increase it by one capsule every three or four days until your symptoms have resolved or until you feel groggy in the morning (that means you've taken too much). Then back down a capsule or two. The maximum dose of progesterone is about 200 mg or eight capsules per night. There is a non-compounded bio-identical form of progesterone called Prometrium, but it only comes in 100 mg or 200 mg capsules. Some of my patients also react to the fillers in there, but it is an option for those who don't have access to a provider prescribe compounded hormones.

If you don't have access to a medical provider, consider the supplement Progonol, a fermented plant derived progesterone cream derived from wild yam. You ramp-up by 1/8 tsp every three or four days.

Once you have found the right dose for you, check your levels in urine.

Testosterone Therapy

For testosterone treatment in women, I recommend 1 mg in 0.1 ml of cream. If that doesn't resolve your testosterone deficiency symptoms, then use the Testosterone Ramp-Up. This entails increasing by 0.1 ml every week up to a maximum of about 0.5 ml (5 mg). In women, signs of testosterone excess include excessive hair growth and aggression.

In men, I recommend starting with 50 mg per day in 0.1 ml of cream applied to the anus. If that doesn't resolve your symptoms, then increase weekly by 50 mg until your symptoms resolve, you get symptoms of testosterone excess, or you achieve the maximum of 300 mg. Testosterone can convert to other hormones that you don't want, so you'll need to check these regularly. They are dihydrotestosterone (DHT) and estrogen. You can check these in blood. If these levels are increasing, then discontinue or decrease the testosterone, or use supplements and medications to inhibit the conversion.

If you are not responding to testosterone therapy, you may need to remedy the *usual suspects* first.

Hormone Treatment Tips

The Ramp-Up protocols require you to keep close track of how you are feeling day to day so that you know when you've reached the right dose for you. I recommend that you track your symptoms in a journal or using the Symptom Calendar in the member area of our website (fixyourfatigue.org/members). Remember, once you sign up, all the resources are free.

Make sure you bring the Symptom Calendar with you to the follow-up appointments with your healthcare provider so that you can convey the change (or lack thereof) in your symptoms. If you need to make a change to your hormones, change only one hormone at a time so you can understand how your symptoms respond.

Also, make sure you always bring in your hormone prescriptions when you need a refill. Sometimes what the provider wants and what the compounding pharmacy thinks they mean need clarification.

I generally start BHRT without laboratory testing, since the symptoms of the deficiencies are unique. There is not a lot of crossover between the hormones, especially when dealing with menopause and andropause.

IMPORTANT: Working with a medical professional, preferably a provider trained in functional medicine, is always advised for treating the nuances of your condition. This type of practitioner can assist you with laboratory testing and interpretation of the results, as well as customize your treatments and monitor your progress to make sure you're proceeding safely.

Summary

Imbalances in sex hormones are much more common than you might think and can cause fatigue in both men and women. Besides fatigue, sex hormone imbalances can produce many signs and symptoms, including (but not limited to) hot flashes, premenstrual symptoms, low libido, erectile dysfunction, infertility, polycystic ovaries, mood instability and sleep disturbances. Bringing hormones into balance can dramatically improve your energy and quality of life, and can ease the transition through menopause and andropause.

Bringing your sex hormones into balance has other health benefits, including lowering your risk for heart attack, stroke, and Alzheimer's disease.

Hormone levels can be assessed using blood, urine, and saliva testing, and each has appropriate applications. Hormone imbalances today are complicated by stress and overwhelmed adrenals as well as exposure to xenoestrogens (estrogen disrupting chemicals), which are present all around us. Your adrenals and thyroid must be regulated before the ovaries or testes can function optimally.

I've had success correcting sex hormone imbalances with bio-identical estrogen, progesterone, and testosterone, using a combination of oral and topical forms. This is useful with menopause and andropause.

The Plan

1. Always start low, go slow, mimic nature, and measure. Use herbs when you can and if you need prescriptions, use the minimum amount needed. Use topical BHRT except for progesterone.

2. Treat based on symptoms and confirm with laboratory testing.

<u>For Symptoms of Estrogen Deficiency</u>

1. Start FemmenessencePro (maca) Ramp-Up:

   a. Week 1: 1 capsule in the morning.

   b. Week 2: 1 capsule in the morning, 1 capsule at noon.

   c. Week 3: 2 capsule in the morning, 1 capsule at noon.

   d. Week 4: 2 capsules in the morning, 2 capsules at noon.

e. If you are experiencing nausea or a dull headache, decrease to the previous dose for one more week, then reattempt.

f. Our online store does not have this product, so you need to get it here: https://www.npscript.com/drevanhirsch/femmeness encepro/NH0001PAR

g. If this doesn't take care of your symptoms after two months, proceed to the next step.

2. Start Ostaderm-V cream, 1/8 tsp every night applied to skin creases. Increase by 1/8 tsp every week until your symptoms resolve. If you experience breast tenderness, you've gone too far, and you need to back down by 1/8 tsp.

    a. Once you get the dose you need, then add in progesterone (or Progonol).

    b. Our online store does not have this product, so you need to get it here: https://www.npscript.com/drevanhirsch/ostader m-v-1-1-8/BE0014PAR

    c. If you need more control of your dose in a smaller amount of cream, then proceed to the next step.

    d. Start compounded Bi-est (80% estriol, 20% estradiol) 0.5 mg in 0.2 ml. Then increase using the Estrogen Ramp-Up by 0.1 ml every week until symptoms resolve. If you experience breast tenderness, you've gone too far, and you need to back down 0.1 ml. Once you get the dose you need of Bi-est, then add in progesterone 20 mg to keep things in balance if you're not going to use oral progesterone. Consider adding in testosterone as well. Recheck urine levels and uterine ultrasounds once symptoms resolve and then annually.

For Symptoms of Estrogen Excess

Start vitex (chasteberry) 1 capsule two times per day and increase up to 2 capsules two times per day as needed for more support. Consider only taking it when you have symptoms if you don't need it every day.

For Symptoms of Progesterone Deficiency

1. Start FemmenessencePro (maca) Ramp-Up:

   a. Week 1: 1 capsule in the morning.

   b. Week 2: 1 capsule in the morning, 1 capsule at noon.

   c. Week 3: 2 capsule in the morning, 1 capsule at noon.

   d. Week 4: 2 capsules in the morning, 2 capsules at noon.

   e. If you are experiencing nausea or a dull headache, decrease to the previous dose for one more week, then reattempt.

   f. Our online store does not have this product, so you need to get it here: https://www.npscript.com/drevanhirsch/femmenessencepro/NH0001PAR

   g. If this doesn't take care of your symptoms after two months, stop taking it and proceed to the next step.

2. Start Progonol cream, 1/8 tsp every night applied to skin creases (back of the knees, etc.). Increase by 1/8 tsp every three days until your symptoms resolve or until you are groggy in the mornings. Then back off by 1/8 tsp to avoid the grogginess.

   a. Our online store does not have this product, so you need to get it here: https://www.npscript.com/drevanhirsch/progonol-cream/BE0028PAR

   b. If you need more control of your dose in a smaller amount of cream, or you want it orally, then proceed to the next step.

3. Start compounded progesterone oral 25mg capsules. Take 1 capsule at night and increase using the Progesterone Ramp-Up by 1 capsule every three days until your symptoms resolve or until you are groggy in the mornings. Then back off by 1 capsule to avoid the grogginess. Alternatively, you can use a topical cream and put 25 mg in 0.2 ml and increase by 0.2 ml at the same rate. Recheck urine levels once your symptoms resolve and then annually.

For Symptoms of Testosterone Deficiency in Women

1. Start FemmenessencePro (maca) Ramp-Up:

   a. Week 1: 1 capsule in the morning.

   b. Week 2: 1 capsule in the morning, 1 capsule at noon.

   c. Week 3: 2 capsule in the morning, 1 capsule at noon.

   d. Week 4: 2 capsules in the morning, 2 capsules at noon.

e. If you are experiencing nausea or a dull headache, decrease to the previous dose for one more week, then reattempt.

f. Our online store does not have this product, so you need to get it here: https://www.npscript.com/drevanhirsch/femmenessencepro/NH0001PAR

g. If this doesn't take care of your symptoms after two months, proceed to the next step.

2. Start compounded testosterone 1 mg in 0.1 ml. Increase using the Testosterone Ramp-Up by 0.1 ml every week until you achieve symptom relief. Max dose recommended is 5 mg (or 0.5 ml). Recheck blood or urine levels once your symptoms resolve and then annually.

Once you have determined the proper dosing individually of all the hormones you need, you can then combine them into one cream to save money and for convenience.

<u>For Symptoms of Testosterone Deficiency in Men</u>

1. Start RevolutionPro (maca) Ramp-Up:

a. Week 1: 1 capsule in the morning

b. Week 2: 1 capsule in the morning, 1 capsule at noon.

c. Week 3: 2 capsule in the morning, 1 capsule at noon

d. Week 4: 2 capsule in the morning, 2 capsules at noon.

e. If you are experiencing nausea or a dull headache, decrease to the previous dose for one more week, then reattempt.

f. Our online store does not have this product, so you need to get it here: https://www.npscript.com/revolutionpro/NH0002P AR

g. If this doesn't take care of your symptoms after two months, proceed to the next step

2. Start compounded testosterone 50 mg in 0.2 ml. Increase by 0.1 ml every week until you achieve symptom relief. Max dose recommended is 300 mg. Recheck blood or urine levels once your symptoms resolve and then annually.

Action Steps

1. Order the new supplements discussed in this chapter and start the ramp-up! You can find the maca products, progonol, and ostaderm-V here: https://www.npscript.com/drevanhirsch (not our usual online store).

2. The vitex can be found in our usual online store here in the Sex Hormone Support category: us.fullscript.com/welcome/drhirsch

3. Add your new supplements to your Treatment Schedule & Calendar (free in the member area at fixyourfatigue.org/members)

4. Set alarms on your phone to remind you to take your supplements

5. Track your symptoms on your Symptom Calendar (free in the member area)

6. Stop drinking from water bottles to decrease xenoestrogens

7. Questions? Ask people in our Facebook group (fb.com/groups/fixyourfatigue) questions like these:

   a. *Which form of progesterone do you like the best? Oral or topical?*

   b. *How long did it take you to ramp up on your Ostaderm-V or Bi-est before you got to the right dose?*

   c. *What benefits have you seen with BHRT? Any side effects?*

8. Continue to implement the lifestyle changes you have made and the treatments since then.

9. Congratulations on completing another chapter!

10. Get ready to Fix Your Nutrients in the next chapter!

Chapter 12:
Fix Your Nutrients

*L*eigh *couldn't sleep, her energy was low, and her memory wasn't working right. She couldn't find the right words at the right times. She also had a mild tingling sensation in her legs occasionally, and she was a vegan. She had a vitamin B12 deficiency.*

Background

There was a time when nutrient deficiencies were not an issue for humans. But because of changes in our diet and stress, we must replace nutrients. Otherwise, we suffer the consequences of ill health, including fatigue.

The top five nutrient deficiencies I've identified among my fatigue patients are:

- Vitamin B12

- Vitamin D

- Magnesium

- Folate (vitamin B9)

- Iron

The Causes of Nutrient Deficiencies

Nutrients become deficient when:

1. **The foods that contain them are not consumed in sufficient quantity**. The Standard American Diet

(SAD) consists largely of processed foods that are high in sugar and flour and low in nutritional content. This is the main diet consumed in the United States. Whole foods are the solution.

2. **The foods that used to contain them are stripped of their nutrients**. Plant foods absorb their nutrients from the soil. If the soil has been stripped of its nutrients by poor crop rotation and lack of attention to the health of the soil, the quantity and quality of nutrients in the plant will be lacking.

3. **The foods that contain the nutrients are not broken down sufficiently by the body**. Nothing shuts down digestion faster than stress. This stress response may result from a mental, emotional, physical or energetic stressor. These stressors decrease the production of stomach acid and consequently the breakdown of food.

4. **The body does not absorb them**. The stressors mentioned above also decrease the production of digestive enzymes, stomach acid, and bile salts. This leads to poor absorption of the nutrients. Some physical stressors cause inflammation in the gut. They include food allergies, genetically modified organisms (GMOs), pesticides, herbicides, parasites, and autoimmunity.

5. **The need for the nutrient exceeds the amount that is being consumed**. A stressor or a genetic predisposition may create a greater demand for nutrients.

6. **There is a genetic predisposition.** Some genetic issues lead to lower levels of nutrient absorption.

I'm now going to go through each of the nutrients mentioned above and discuss symptoms, testing, and treatment.

Vitamin B12

A vitamin B12 deficiency can cause fatigue in many people, so it's one of the most important nutrient levels to check. It is involved in many reactions in the body, including the normal functioning of the brain, nervous system, and red blood cells.

Symptoms

Vitamin B12 deficiency can lead to:

- Fatigue

- Depression

- Anxiety

- Insomnia

- Neuropathy (nerve pain or dysfunction)

- Cognitive issues

- Brain fog

- Memory loss

Testing

There are several ways to test for vitamin B12. The most common and easiest way is via a blood sample. The following includes the laboratory tests that I use to assess vitamin B12 levels in the body and the optimal ranges.

Vitamin B12	1500-2000 pg/ml
Homocysteine	5-7 umol/L
Mean Corpuscular Volume (MCV)	90-96 fL

What Causes B12 Deficiency?

There are several reasons why you may be deficient in vitamin B12.

1. **You may not be eating enough foods high in B12.** Vitamin B12 is found primarily in red meat and eggs. If you have a deficiency, you may be under-consuming those foods. This problem is especially common in my vegan and vegetarian patients.

2. **Insufficient stomach acid.** A significant amount of stomach acid is required to properly break down food, free up B12, and release a glycoprotein called intrinsic factor from the lining of the stomach. Once liberated, intrinsic factor will bind to B12 and be absorbed in the terminal ileum, the third part (last section) of the small intestine. Vitamin B12 absorption can go awry anywhere in that process. If stomach acid is inadequate, intrinsic factor cannot be liberated from the lining of the stomach, so B12 cannot be absorbed.

3. **Autoimmunity.** Pernicious anemia is an autoimmune condition in which antibodies bind to intrinsic factor, preventing B12 absorption. This B12 deficiency requires ongoing B12 shots.

4. **Increased need**. If the body is using up a lot of B12 because of an intense detoxification process or stress, B12 deficiency can develop. Vitamin B12 and folate play essential roles in methylation (phase two detoxification in the liver). Vitamin B12 is necessary for converting homocysteine to methionine, which is the first step in that process. Consequently, if your vitamin B12 levels are low, detoxification will be compromised.

5. **Genetic predisposition**. If you have genetic variations in your MTHFR, MTR, or MTRR genes (found in methylation), your body requires more vitamin B12 to detoxify, and you will require supplementation.

6. **Excessive B vitamin intake**. If you are taking too much folate or other B vitamins, they can push the vitamin B12 out of the body and cause a deficiency. The converse is also true, if you take too much B12, you can get deficiencies in other B vitamins.

7. **Stress**. During times of physical, mental, emotional, and energetic stress you will require more vitamin B12.

What is Methylation?

Methylation is a biochemical process that is essential for the proper functioning of the body's systems. It helps repair your DNA (genetic material) on a daily basis, it controls homocysteine (which can damage blood vessels), it supports detoxification (the removal of waste products from the body), and it helps to maintain mood and keep inflammation in check. When methylation isn't working right, you have a greater risk for fatigue, osteoporosis, diabetes, cervical cancer, colon cancer, lung cancer, depression, dementia, and stroke.

And you may be at higher risk for cardiovascular disease. Optimal levels of B vitamins and other nutrients keep methylation running smoothly.

You can learn more about your genetics by ordering a lab kit at 23andme.com and importing this data into geneticgenie.org.

Vitamin B12 Treatment

Once you have the appropriate vitamin B12 tests, you can interpret your levels and treat.

1. Vitamin B12 levels 1500 pg/mL or above: Ideal

2. Vitamin B12 levels below 550 pg/mL: *This is very low*, warranting vitamin B12 injections or very high doses of oral B12. I've had success treating my patients with 10,000 mcg per day sublingual (under the tongue) or 2,000 mcg injections of B12 every other day for two months. After two months, we decrease the frequency to twice a week for one month, and then once a week. Patients typically need to continue once-a-week injections for a while.

3. Vitamin B12 levels between 550 and 1500 pg/mL: I recommend 5,000 mcg per day of a sublingual B12.

4. A homocysteine level greater than 7 indicates that B12, folate, or thyroid is deficient. This is because homocysteine is processed by B12 and folate. When enough B12 and folate are present, homocysteine levels will drop as homocysteine is converted to methionine. As you treat these deficiencies, your homocysteine level will move into the normal range. An elevated level of homocysteine is also associated with an increased risk of a heart attack, stroke, and Alzheimer's disease.

5. A MCV level greater than 96 indicates that your red blood cells are larger than they should be because you have a B12, folate, or thyroid deficiency. As you treat these deficiencies, your MCV level will move into the normal range.

Choosing the Right Form of B12 for You

As always, I recommend starting at a low dose of B12 and working up over time until the correct level is reached and your symptoms are resolved.

There are many forms of B12, but not every form is appropriate for you. Ideally, we would all be able to tolerate methylated B12. This form of B12 is the best form for absorption and utilization in the body. However, I have seen many cases when methylated B12 makes a patient feel worse. This is due to individual genetic variations. If I do not know someone's genetic profile, I will default to the hydroxyB12 form to avoid any reactions. This form works very well and is very well tolerated.

Vitamin B12 also must be balanced with the other B vitamins. I balance the B vitamins with a good multi or B-complex, making sure to include methylfolate. I've witnessed significant improvements in my patients' sleep, energy, mental function, depression, and anxiety when their vitamin B12 levels are restored. Don't underestimate the importance of B12!

The Sunshine Vitamin

Before the year 2000, very few physicians thought about checking their patients' vitamin D levels. Now that testing is widely available, laboratory data has revealed just how prevalent vitamin D deficiency is in the United States. Dr. Michael Holick, a leading vitamin D researcher and author of

The Vitamin D Solution, estimates that 50 percent of the general population is at risk for vitamin D deficiency, and this percentage rises in higher-risk populations such as the elderly and those with darker skin.

Vitamin D is unique because your body turns it into a hormone, which is sometimes called "activated vitamin D" or "calcitriol."

Many of your body's organs are dependent on vitamin D for proper function, including your thyroid gland and pancreas. Vitamin D has wide-ranging health benefits, from reducing high blood pressure and heart disease risk to preventing infections, immune system modulation, metabolism, and DNA repair.

When our skin is exposed directly to the sun, vitamin D is converted into its active form. Consequently, vitamin D deficiency is more common in people who live in areas with less direct sunlight. In the higher latitudes where the sun is at a lower angle, there are more clouds, and the air is cooler, people's levels of vitamin D are lower. Having a medical practice in Olympia, Washington, I see a lot of vitamin D deficiency. However, somewhat surprisingly, recent research has shown vitamin D deficiencies are just as prevalent in hotter climates, such as Arizona, because people have concerns about sun exposure, so they limit their outdoor activities and always wear sunscreen. Today's predominantly indoor, sedentary lifestyles undoubtedly are contributing to lower vitamin D levels.

Symptoms

Because vitamin D is involved in so many biological processes, a deficiency can produce wide-ranging symptoms, including but not limited to:

- Fatigue

- Anxiety and depression

- Seasonal mood changes (Seasonal Affective Disorder, or SAD)

- Chronic pain and fibromyalgia

- Pain and dysfunction from autoimmunity

Autoimmunity

Vitamin D's natural immune modulation is especially strong at the higher doses (20,000 IU per day). It stimulates T-regulatory helper cells to balance out Th1 and Th2 immunity. These components of the immune system are out of balance during autoimmunity. Dosing vitamin D at 20,000 IU per day, however, is not advised for everyone. There is some new research to suggest that excessive dosing can be detrimental to our health.

Testing

The best way to determine your vitamin D level is with a blood test. I recommend testing for 25-hydroxyvitamin D. Your ideal level will be between 60 and 100 ng/mL.

Treatment

The best way to optimize your vitamin D levels is by spending time outdoors with direct sun exposure. Of course, that's not always possible depending on the climate where you live. If natural sun exposure is not possible for you, oral vitamin D supplementation is a good option.

When someone's vitamin D level is:

1. Below 60 ng/mL, I recommend 5,000 IU of vitamin D daily.

2. Below 20 ng/mL, I recommend 10,000 IU daily. A few patients require up to 25,000 IU per day to get their blood level to rise.

People who require very high doses of vitamin D to get their levels up to 60 ng/mL frequently have a vitamin D receptor (VDR) genetic variation that inhibits the vitamin D uptake into the cells. In this situation, your cells can be "opened up" with the herbs rosemary and sage. You can cook with those herbs daily or take them in pill form; either is helpful.

You can find out if you have this gene and others through 23andme.com. When you get the results, go to geneticgenie.org and follow the prompts to transfer your data from 23andme.com to view a report.

How to Safely Get Enough Vitamin D from the Sun

Natural sunshine is the absolute best way to get your vitamin D. According to the Vitamin D Council, your skin can produce about 20,000 IU (International Units) of vitamin D after twenty minutes of sun exposure.

If you have access to natural sunshine, it's best to expose as much of your skin as possible. The duration of exposure depends on many factors, such as pigmentation, age, antioxidant levels, latitude, cloud cover, etc. Dr. Holick, author of *The Vitamin D Solution*, recommends exposing your skin until it turns the lightest shade of pink. This is typically about *half the time it would take you to get a mild sunburn.*

After exposure to direct sunlight, avoid washing your skin (especially with soap), as there is some evidence that the oils on your skin's surface need time to be absorbed for proper vitamin D production to occur. For more on this, refer to the blog article entitled "Washing Away Vitamin D" by John Cannell, MD, founder of the Vitamin D Council.

I recommend skin cover with clothing and a hat after you have exposed your skin for twenty minutes. Most sunscreen is toxic, so I don't recommend it unless it is deemed safe by the Environmental Working Group at ewg.org/skindeep. This is the site I recommend for assessing the health impact of your household products and cosmetics. We will discuss this in more detail in the chapter on chemicals.

Magnesium: The Wonder Mineral

Magnesium deficiency is another common cause of fatigue. This mineral is involved in more than five hundred different enzymatic reactions in the body, so it is incredibly important.

Symptoms

If you're not getting enough magnesium, you may experience:

- Constipation

- Muscle pain

- Muscle spasms

- Muscle cramping

- Insomnia

- Adrenal dysfunction

- Fatigue

Several of these conditions will lead to fatigue.

People require different amounts of magnesium depending on what's going on in their lives at any particular time. For example, your magnesium reserves may fall due to an increased demand by the adrenals during stressful times.

Here are some examples of magnesium's many functions in the body:

- **Adrenal support**: Magnesium is incredibly nourishing for the adrenals. It provides support for the enzymes that make adrenal hormones. During times of stress, the adrenals make more stress hormones, and magnesium becomes depleted.

- **Detoxification**: Magnesium opens up detoxification pathways in the methylation cycle.

- **Constipation**: Magnesium treats constipation by relaxing smooth muscle (in the intestines) and allowing the stool to move through more easily. Use a non-chelated form (usually citrate) for this laxative effect.

- **Sleep support**: Magnesium is a great sleep aid because it relaxes the central nervous system. Use a chelated form for better absorption.

- **Muscle relaxation**: Magnesium is also a great muscle relaxer. Calcium causes muscles to contract, and magnesium causes them to relax. In addition to oral supplementation, I recommend Epsom salt (magnesium sulfate) baths, as long as you can tolerate sulfur. If you cannot, take magnesium chloride baths.

Testing

Magnesium deficiency can be tested in blood serum, red blood cells, or in urine. For convenience, I recommend serum blood testing and a level of magnesium 2.3-2.5 mg/dL for optimal function.

Treatment

There are many forms of magnesium. If you have a magnesium deficiency and you're not constipated, I recommend you take magnesium chelate because the chelated form is the best absorbed. Start with capsules or powder, 250 mg per night, and increase with a Magnesium Ramp-Up by one capsule every three nights until you get soft stools. This is considered your bowel tolerance. Just about everybody will get diarrhea if they consume enough magnesium. I want you to consume as much as you can until you get to that point, and then you can lower the dose by one capsule so that you don't have diarrhea. The goal is to have soft, well-formed stools one or two times a day while absorbing as much magnesium as you can.

If you are constipated, use magnesium citrate or magnesium oxide. You will get the laxative effect sooner than with the chelated form. Constipation causes the recycling of toxins from your intestines back into your blood stream. This increases the toxicity in your body and can cause (and worsen) fatigue symptoms.

Of course, consuming more magnesium-rich foods is always important. Here are five foods that will give you the most magnesium:

- Sprouts, including mung bean, sunflower, pea shoots, etc. Sprouts are little nutritional powerhouses containing twenty to thirty times the nutrients of their adult veggie counterparts. When a seed starts to sprout, minerals such as calcium and magnesium bind to proteins in the seed, which makes the minerals and the protein more readily available and usable in your body.

- Dark leafy greens, including spinach, collards, kale, and chard. Spinach and chard deliver 157 mg of magnesium per cup.

- Pumpkin seeds are extremely high in magnesium: 92 mg per 1/8 cup; other nuts and seeds include almonds, sunflower seeds, Brazil nuts, cashews, pine nuts, flaxseed, and pecans.

- Dark chocolate will give you 95 mg of magnesium per square!

  Notes on chocolate: If you crave chocolate, you usually have a magnesium deficiency. Please avoid chocolate if it makes you feel worse. Pay attention to how you sleep when you eat chocolate; the caffeine may affect your quality of sleep.

- Black beans contain 60 mg of magnesium per ½ cup.

Folate (Vitamin B9)

Folate, also known vitamin B9, is one of many essential vitamins needed for copying and synthesizing DNA, producing new cells, and supporting nerve and immune functions. A water-soluble B vitamin, folate is naturally present in some foods, added to others, and available as a dietary supplement in the form of folic acid.

Studies show that a diet high in folate-rich foods can help prevent cancer, heart disease, birth defects, anemia, and cognitive decline.

Symptoms

Symptoms of folate deficiency include:

- Memory loss

- Headaches

- Decreased libido

- Detoxification problems

- Neuropathy (nerve pain/dysfunction)

- Chemical sensitivity

- Poor immune function

- Frequently getting sick

- Fatigue

- Constipation

- Bloating

- Developmental problems during pregnancy and infancy

- Anemia

- Canker sores in the mouth

- Swollen tongue

- Irritability

- Premature hair graying

- Pale skin

Folate vs. Folic Acid

It is common for lay people and medical professional alike to confuse folate with folic acid, as many use the terms interchangeably. But there are important distinctions. Folate refers to the group of water-soluble B-vitamins that naturally occur in foods, also known as vitamin B9. Folic acid is the oxidized synthetic compound used in some dietary supplements and commercial food fortification. Several studies have reported adverse effects from the presence of folic acid in the blood from folic acid supplements or fortified foods. Most of us do not metabolize it well. In fact, nearly half the population has a genetic variation in the MTHFR gene that prevents them from receiving benefit from folic acid.

The causes of folate deficiency include not eating enough folate-rich foods and an increased need for detoxification processes.

Testing

Folate levels are tested by measuring red blood cell (RBC) folate in blood. Optimal levels are 1500-2000 ng/ml.

Treatment

I treat folate deficiency by prescribing the methylated form of folate: methylfolate. In most cases, 1 to 2 mg per day will achieve the recommended blood levels. If a patient has depression, anxiety, a genetic predisposition for detoxification problems, an increased risk for cardiovascular disease, schizophrenia, Alzheimer's, or Parkinson's, I will increase the folate slowly as tolerated up to a maximum dose of 15 mg per day.

As mentioned, B12 and folate play huge roles in methylation (phase two detoxification). The first step in methylation is the conversion of homocysteine to methionine. Vitamin B12 and folate are used as enzymes for this pathway. If a genetic issue compromises this pathway, taking larger doses of B12 and folate can help move things along. Remember, it's critical to balance folate, B12, and all of the other B vitamins, so adding a good quality B-complex or multivitamin is a good idea.

You can also increase the amount of folate you are consuming in your diet. Five foods rich in folate are:

- **Leafy greens**: Spinach, endive, romaine lettuce, mustard greens, turnip greens. Spinach: 1687 mcg per 200 calorie serving. Sprout those seeds! (See the bit about sprouts under magnesium-rich foods, above)

- **Asparagus**: 1600 mcg per 200 calorie serving

- **Broccoli**: 900 mcg per 200 calorie serving

- **Beans**: Adzuki, mung, cranberry, pinto, fava, kidney, lima, garbanzo. Adzuki: 378 mcg per 200 calorie serving

- **Boysenberries**: 252 mcg per 200 calorie serving

Iron

Iron deficiency is the most common nutritional deficiency in the U.S., according to the Centers for Disease Control (CDC), with almost 10 percent of women being considered iron deficient! Iron is an essential nutrient that supports many functions throughout the body every single day, including the transport of oxygen throughout the blood.

Iron helps metabolize proteins and plays a role in the production of hemoglobin in red blood cells. Hemoglobin carries oxygen from your lungs to the rest of your body. Consequently, if you are iron-deficient, you may be oxygen-deficient as well. Many women feel fatigued during their menstrual cycles because of this phenomenon. Iron deficiency is a common cause of fatigue.

Most of the 3 to 4 grams of elemental iron present within the body is carried in your red blood cells as hemoglobin. The remaining iron is stored in the liver, spleen, and bone marrow.

Symptoms

Symptoms of iron deficiency include the following:

- Anemia

- Fatigue

- Pale or yellowing skin

- Shortness of breath

- Heart palpitations

- Muscle weakness

- Appetite changes

- Sleep problems

- Cough

- Memory and cognitive impairment

- Mood changes

Causes of Iron Deficiency

The following can cause iron deficiency:

1. Menstrual cycle

2. Not eating enough foods rich in iron

3. Poor iron absorption

4. Infections and biofilm deposition

Causes of Iron Excess

Iron excess is most commonly caused by a genetic condition called hemochromatosis that causes the deposition of iron into different organs.

Testing

To test for iron deficiency, I recommend the following laboratory tests. Please be aware that none of these tests can make the diagnosis alone; it is the combination of them that shows us the true picture:

- **Total Iron Binding Capacity (TIBC):** The TIBC tells how strongly the body is binding to the iron. If iron levels are low, the body will bind to it more tightly. If this number is above 400, there is a high likelihood of iron deficiency.

- **Ferritin**: Ferritin is a protein that binds to iron and stores it. I recommend a level of 40-50. If your level is less than 40, you may be iron-deficient. Ferritin can be falsely elevated during times of inflammation and infections.

- **Mean Corpuscular Volume (MCV):** If the MCV is less than 90, this indicates red blood cells that are too small (also called microcytic anemia). This is a good test for iron deficiency.

To test for iron excess (or overload), you will want to determine the following:

- **An elevated level of ferritin.** A ferritin level above 80 may be indicative of hemochromatosis, so the genetic markers need to be run.

- **Hemochromatosis markers**. These genetic markers look at iron overload in the body. If the results are heterozygous (this means that one gene has the marker for it and one gene does not), you *may* have the condition. If the results are homozygous (both genes have the marker), you *do* have the condition.

Treating Iron Deficiency

First, try to increase your iron levels from consuming more meat, leafy green, veggies and spinach. If you still need more iron, start supplementing with elemental iron.

Treating Iron Excess

There are two ways to treat iron excess in the body. The first is with therapeutic phlebotomy (blood-letting) or donating blood on a regular basis. You can donate blood through your local blood bank every six weeks. This may be enough to resolve the overload, or you may need to be drawn more frequently by your blood bank or local hospital with an order from your provider. Trial and error will determine how much should be withdrawn and how often to do so. I have had some patients who require phlebotomy every two weeks, and some need it every eight weeks. If you feel worse afterward, and it takes a while for you to recover, decrease the frequency of your phlebotomy.

The other technique is to push iron oxide out of the organs by taking a lot of magnesium oxide.

Summary

Five particular nutrient deficiencies play significant roles in fatigue: Vitamin B12, vitamin D, magnesium, folate, and iron.

In addition to fatigue, vitamin B12 deficiencies may contribute to mood issues, insomnia, cognitive problems, and neuropathy. Low B12 may result from inadequate consumption of B12-rich foods, problems with digestion or absorption, high demand for B12, or autoimmune processes. Deficiencies can be treated using oral/sublingual B12 or injections.

Vitamin D deficiency is common in the United States due to insufficient sun exposure. Many organs in the body are dependent on vitamin D for proper function, so blood levels should be checked regularly. Low vitamin D may cause fatigue, depression, anxiety, chronic pain, and autoimmunity. Levels can be boosted using an oral supplement or increased safe sun exposure.

Magnesium is involved in more than five hundred different enzymatic reactions in the body. If you're not getting enough magnesium, you may experience constipation, muscle pain or dysfunction, insomnia, detoxification problems, adrenal dysfunction, and fatigue. My preferred form is magnesium chelate because of its higher absorption rate.

Folate deficiency can cause problems with mood, detoxification, and chemical sensitivity. For folate deficiency, I use methyl folate (also known as L-5-MTHF). B12 and folate play significant roles in methylation and phase 2 detoxification, so it's important to pay attention to them and to balance the other B vitamins with a good quality B-complex or multi.

My experience has shown that correcting deficiencies in vitamin B12, vitamin D, magnesium, folate, and iron will make a significant improvement in your recovery from chronic fatigue.

The Plan

<u>For vitamin B12 deficiency</u>

1. Start Activated B-12 Guard (Vitamin B12) 2 tabs under the tongue each morning.

2. Start Innate One Daily 1 tablet per day for B-vitamin balance, vitamin and mineral support.

3. Goal: Blood levels should be 1500-2000.

<u>For vitamin D deficiency</u>

1. Start Vitamin D Supreme 5,000-10,000 IU per day depending lab testing.

2. Goal: Blood levels should be 60-100

<u>For magnesium deficiency without constipation</u>

1. Start Magnesium chelate 1 cap per night and increase by 1 cap every three nights until soft stools, then back down by 1 capsule to avoid diarrhea. (This is the Magnesium Ramp-Up)

2. Goal: Blood levels above 2.3

<u>For magnesium deficiency with constipation</u>

1. Start Triple Mag (magnesium) 1 cap per night and increase by 1 cap every three nights until soft stools, then back down by 1 capsule to avoid diarrhea. (Magnesium Ramp-Up)

2. Goal: Soft stools, one to two bowel movements per day, and blood levels above 2.3

For folate deficiency

1. Start L-5MTHF (methylfolate) 1mg each morning

2. Goal: Blood levels 1500 2000

For iron deficiency

1. Start Ferrochel (elemental iron) 1 capsule per night. You can take it during the day, but it needs to be taken two hours away from thyroid medication. Watch for stomach irritation and constipation.

2. Goal: Blood levels of ferritin >50, TIBC <400, MCV >90.

For iron excess (Hemochromatosis)

1. Start donating blood every six weeks. If this is helpful, and you want it more frequently, ask your provider to write you an order for a monthly blood draw.

2. Start Magnesium Oxide 1 cap per night and increase by 1 cap every three nights until soft stools, then back down by 1 capsule to avoid diarrhea. (Magnesium Ramp-Up)

3. Goal: Soft stools, one to two bowel movements per day, blood levels above 2.3, ferritin <80

Action Steps

1. Order the new supplements discussed in this chapter and start the Magnesium Ramp-Up! You can find them under the Nutrient Deficiencies category in our online store here: us.fullscript.com/welcome/drhirsch

2. Add your new supplements to your Treatment Schedule & Calendar (free at fixyourfatigue.org/members)

3. Set alarms on your phone to remind you to take your supplements

4. Track your symptoms on your Symptom Calendar (free in the member area)

5. Questions? Ask people in our Facebook group (fb.com/groups/fixyourfatigue) questions like these:

    a. *How much magnesium did it take you to get to bowel tolerance?*

    b. *Who else is seeing better sleep since starting B12?*

6. Continue to implement the lifestyle changes you have made and the treatments since then.

7. Congratulations on completing another chapter!

8. Get ready to Fix Your Mitochondria in the next chapter.

Chapter 13:
Fix Your Mitochondria

*A*lan had mold toxicity, mercury toxicity, and Lyme disease. His energy improved as we treated each of these components, but once these issues were gone, he didn't have the energy I thought he should. I did some more testing and found that his mitochondria needed repair. Once we fixed his mitochondria, his energy improved significantly.

Background

Mitochondria are the body's energy generators. They take nutrients and convert them into adenosine triphosphate (ATP) in the cells to regulate metabolism through a process called the Krebs cycle, which is what humans use as energy to perform the many various tasks and functions in the body. They are necessary for proper functioning of the heart, liver, kidneys, GI tract, brain, and nervous system. Without healthy, functioning mitochondria, we can't expect to function at full capacity.

Diet determines the energy made in the mitochondria. If we do not have an adequate supply of healthy fats (the preferred energy source for mitochondria), carbohydrates, and proteins to feed into stage 1 of the Krebs cycle, we will experience fatigue.

Mitochondria have their own DNA, or genetic material. This DNA will get damaged by nutrient deficiencies, toxins, and some pharmaceutical medications. These toxins include the *usual suspects* – heavy metals, chemicals, mold, infections, emotions, electromagnetic frequencies, and allergies. This is very important to note because often providers will treat the *usual suspects* to resolution and wonder why the patient's fatigue is not gone. It's because the mitochondria need repair!

Once the DNA is damaged, it can no longer function properly. Less ATP will be produced, and fatigue will result.

According to the United Mitochondrial Disease Foundation, mitochondria are responsible for creating more than 90 percent of the energy needed to sustain the human body, but about 75 percent of their job is dedicated to other important cellular processes *besides* energy production. These include growth and development from the time of infancy, bodily functions like digestion, cognitive processes, and maintaining cardiovascular/heartbeat rhythms.

It is important to differentiate between mitochondrial diseases and mitochondrial dysfunction. Mitochondrial diseases are genetic variations and lead to much more serious illnesses. Mitochondrial dysfunction is more mild and repairable.

Symptoms

Symptoms of mitochondrial dysfunction can manifest in different ways and vary in intensity depending on the individual and the organs affected. Some common symptoms and signs include:

- Fatigue

- Loss of motor control, balance, and coordination

- Muscle aches, weakness, and pains

- Digestive problems and gastrointestinal disorders

- Cardiovascular problems and heart disease

- Diabetes and other hormonal disorders

- Vision loss and other visual problems

- Hormonal disorders including a lack of testosterone or estrogen

- Higher susceptibility to infections

Testing

We can test for mitochondrial dysfunction by looking at a number of markers: glutathione levels (serum), GGT, CoQ10, lipid peroxides, 8-OH-dG (8-hydroxy-2'-deoxyguanosine).

Treatment

My initial treatment for mitochondrial dysfunction is to remove the *usual suspects*. This will help the mitochondria start to heal, but additional support is needed to expedite the process. I recommend treating with mitochondrial energy optimizers like:

- D-Ribose

- Acetyl-L-Carnitine

- L-carnitine

- NADH

- Alpha lipoic acid

- Glutathione

- B vitamins

- CoQ10

To support the mitochondria in regeneration and restoration so that it no longer is a cause of your fatigue, I use a product called Mitochondrial NRG. This product combines most of the above components, and I supplement with additional doses of some of them.

A diet rich in fats, proteins, and healthy carbohydrates is also essential for making ATP.

The Plan

1. Remove the *usual suspects*

2. Start Mitochondrial NRG 2 capsules in AM and at noon. This product has a combination of the mitochondrial support listed above.

3. Start Mito-PQQ 1 capsule in AM and at noon. This product increases the number of mitochondria.

4. Start D-Ribose 1 tsp (5 grams) in AM

5. Start the Paleo diet if you haven't already. This diet consists mainly of meat and vegetables. Your plate should be half vegetables, one-quarter meat, and one-quarter starchy vegetable. Eat few to no grains and moderate amounts of fruit.

After a month, if you need additional mitochondrial support, start the following:

1. UBQH (CoQ10) 1 capsule in AM

2. Lipoic Acid 1 capsule two times per day

Action Steps

1. Order the new supplements discussed in this chapter. You can find them under the Mitochondrial Support category in our online store here: us.fullscript.com/welcome/drhirsch

2. Add your new mitochondrial supplements to your Treatment Schedule (fixyourfatigue.org/members)

3. Track your symptoms on the Symptom Calendar

4. Set alarms on your phone to remind you to take your supplements

5. Questions? Ask people in the Facebook group (fb.com/groups/fixyourfatigue) questions like these:

   a. *Who else found that treating mitochondria is the missing step?*

   b. *What symptoms did you have that were relieved with mitochondrial support?*

6. Continue to implement the lifestyle changes you have made and the treatments thus far.

7. Congratulations on completing another chapter! You rock!

8. In the next chapter, it's time for Step III: Remove Toxins!

Step III:
Remove Toxins

Chapter 14:
Fix Your Constipation

For most of my life, I had a bowel movement once a week. I was known for clogging up toilets and became an expert with a plunger. I didn't think there was anything wrong with my bowel habits until I learned in medical school that humans should be stooling daily. It wasn't until I treated my gut infections, dairy allergy, low thyroid, magnesium deficiency, and stress that my constipation resolved.

Background

You may be wondering why constipation is at the beginning of the "Remove the Toxins" section of the book. The first reason is that your detoxification pathways need to be open to proceed through the rest of this section. This requires drinking enough water, getting enough movement, taking B vitamins, eating a clean diet, and having a bowel movement every day.

The second reason is that, unfortunately, when you are constipated, the waste products that are trying to get out of the body are stuck in the gastrointestinal (GI) tract and reabsorbed back into the bloodstream. This increases the total toxic burden on the body and can cause fatigue. So, fixing your constipation will open up your detoxification pathways and decrease the total amount of toxins in your body.

If you have constipation, your digestion is not working right. Unfortunately, many people don't even know they are constipated if they don't have any abdominal pain, bloating or discomfort associated with it. Some people even find it convenient not to have a bowel movement every day!

Causes of Constipation

Stool transit time (the time stool takes to pass through the intestines) can be slowed down (and disrupted) by several mechanisms:

1. **Hypothyroidism**: Low thyroid slows down the metabolic activity of the muscle cells that line the intestines.

2. **Infections in the gut**: Infections will cause inflammation in the gut, which will in turn damage the lining of the GI tract and slow down bowel movements.

3. **Magnesium deficiency**: Magnesium is a natural laxative. It causes the smooth muscle that lines the intestines to relax and allows for more rapid movement of stool through the intestines.

4. **Probiotic imbalance**: There are more bacteria in our intestines than there are cells in our entire body. These bacteria need to be the right kinds to produce the vitamins necessary for optimal function.

5. **Food allergies**: Food allergies cause inflammation leading to the cascade of intestinal damage and inflammation. Gluten, dairy, and other food allergies will produce natural opiates that will slow down gut motility.

6. **Dehydration**: Dehydration makes stool hard and affects its ability to travel through the intestines.

7. **Lack of physical movement**: Physical movement allows for lymph drainage and manually moves stool through the intestines.

8. **Poor diet**: The Standard American Diet (SAD) unfortunately does not consist of enough fruits, vegetables, and fiber to adequately bulk up your stool and move it through your intestines.

9. **Poor positioning**: The best position for stooling is the squatting position because the intestines straighten and allow for better release of stool.

10. **Stress**: mental, emotional, physical (the *usual suspects*), energetic. Nothing shuts down digestion faster than stress. When you are stressed, the digestive juices (enzymes, stomach acid, and bile salts) are not produced the way they should be, and consequently, constipation and other digestive problems can result.

11. **Autoimmunity**: Autoimmune conditions like ulcerative colitis and Crohn's disease can attack the lining of the intestines and cause constipation.

Symptoms

Symptoms of constipation besides fatigue include:

- Not having a bowel movement daily

- Painful bowel movements

- Hemorrhoids

- Pebble-like, hard stools

- Straining on the toilet

- Abdominal pain

- Abdominal bloating

- Foul-smelling gas

- Early satiety – lack of appetite due to a feeling of fullness

Testing

Besides looking at your signs and symptoms, the best way to assess which causes of constipation you have is to run a functional laboratory stool test like the (Metametrix) GI Effects 3-day stool test (DirectLabs.com). This will look at how your digestive juices are functioning (enzymes, stomach acid, bile salts), probiotic balance, the presence of any infections (bacteria, yeast or parasites), and any inflammatory disorders.

Blood testing for thyroid is also in order.

Treatment

My treatment goal for constipation is for you to have two soft and well-formed bowel movements per day. This will help reduce fatigue from the recirculation of toxins due to constipation. I do this by treating all of the cause listed above.

I always start off by recommending enough magnesium to get the laxative effect and achieve daily soft stools. This is called bowel tolerance. This will keep the stool moving and stop the build up of toxins in the body from the constipation. Though magnesium is just a Band-Aid while you figure out other causes of constipation, it is a very safe option. The body can always use more magnesium, since magnesium is involved in 550 different enzymatic reactions in the body and is easily depleted by stress.

I then proceed to test and treat hypothyroidism with the Thyroid Ramp-Up if necessary. If the stool test and symptoms reveal any infections, I treat those following the recommendations in the Fix Your Gut Infections chapter.

I then recommend three to four liters of clean water per day to keep the bowels moving and a diet high in vegetables and fruit and low in grains like the Paleo diet. This will bulk up the stool to help with transport.

I have also found that squatting on the toilet to be very effective. Most of the world squats when they have a bowel movement. This is because squatting straightens and lengthens the intestines to allow for an easier bowel movement.

Further, address stress. This may mean mental, emotional, physical (the *usual suspects*) or energetic stressors. Nothing shuts down digestion faster than stress. When you are stressed, the digestive juices (enzymes, stomach acid, and bile salts) are not produced the way they should be, and consequently, constipation and other digestive problems can result.

Some of my patients may need more intense treatments like daily warm water (or coffee) enemas or pharmaceutical medications like Colace, Dulcolax, and Miralax for short-term use.

Sometimes constipation is caused by gastroparesis. Gastroparesis is a neuropathy, a dysfunction of the nerves responsible for gut motility (movement). Dysfunction in these nerves is often caused by heavy metals, chemicals, molds, and/or infections, and the gastroparesis will not resolve until the cause is treated.

The 5 R Program to Heal Your Gut

As you resolve your constipation, you will want to heal your gut. Follow my gut-healing protocol:

1. **Remove** infections and food allergies.

2. **Replace** digestive juices. Nothing shuts down digestion faster than stress. The body may need reminding of how much and which digestive juices it needs to produce. These juices include:

    a. Betaine HCl: This replaces digestive juices such as hydrochloric acid. Start off with one 700 mg capsule with each meal, and increase every three or four days to a maximum of five capsules per meal. Any time you "feel the warmth," decrease down by one capsule and continue as a slow wean; this retrains the gut to produce enough stomach acid. This is only replaced if your symptoms warrant it.

    b. Pure pancreatic digestive enzymes: One capsule per meal

    c. Ox bile: One capsule per meal. This is only replaced if you have problems with fat absorption (per your stool test results).

3. **Re-inoculate** the gut with probiotics, the good bacteria you need. I recommend 50 billion colony forming units (cfus) per day of a multi-strained probiotic that can survive the stomach acid. I preferred Ther-Biotic Detoxification Support by Klaire Labs or Megaspore.

4. **Repair** leaky gut with:

    a.   Cod liver oil 2 tsp/day

    b.   Glutamine 3 grams/day

    c.   Restore® 1 tsp/meal (restore4life.com)

5. **Replenish** nutrients with the Paleo diet. This means a diet that is whole-foods based and mostly vegetables and meat. Half of your plate should be vegetables, one-quarter meat and one-quarter starchy vegetable (sweet potatoes, beets, carrots and winter squashes). Eat few to no grains and moderate fruit. It's an amazing food plan that increases energy and improves the health of your gut.

Summary

If you have constipation, your digestion is not working right. You need to figure out the causes and remove them to get your digestion back on track. Unfortunately, when you are constipated, the waste products that are trying to get out of the body are stuck in the gastrointestinal (GI) tract and reabsorbed back into the bloodstream. This increases the total toxic burden on the body and can cause fatigue.

The causes of constipation include hypothyroidism, infections in the gut, magnesium deficiency, probiotic imbalance, food allergies, dehydration, lack of physical movement, poor diet, poor positioning, stress, and autoimmunity.

Symptoms associated with constipation include: not having a bowel movement daily, painful bowel movements, hemorrhoids, pebble-like hard stools, straining on the toilet, abdominal pain, abdominal bloating, foul-smelling gas, early satiety – lack of appetite due to a feeling of fullness.

Testing for the causes of constipation includes blood tests for low thyroid and a functional stool test.

Treating constipation should reverse the causes discussed with the goal of having two soft, well-formed bowel movements per day. Once you have resolved the constipation, you will want to heal the gut with the 5 R program.

The Plan

1. Start Triple Mag 1 cap per night and increase according to the Magnesium Ramp-Up by 1 cap every three nights until you achieve one to two soft stools per day. If you get diarrhea, then back down by 1 capsule.

2. Test and treat hypothyroidism if present (see the Fix Your Thyroid chapter).

3. Start (Klaire) Ther-biotic Detox Support or Megaspore probiotic 1 capsule per day.

4. Start Pure Pancreatic Digestive Enzymes 1 capsule per meal.

5. Start squatting on the toilet to position your intestines appropriately. Consider purchasing a squatty potty (squattypotty.com), which is essentially a step stool that slides against the base of a toilet.

6. Start sitting on the toilet at the same time every day to create a habit of daily bowel movements.

7. Start decreasing mental and emotional stress by using Holosync®, meditation, and yoga.

8. Treat any infections in the gut (see the Fix Your Gut Infections chapter).

9. Increase your water intake to three or four liters per day based on your weight (see the Fix Your Water chapter).

10. Increase physical movement by doing ten jumping jacks per day, rebounding, jumping in place, or a seven-minute interval workout. Start low and go slow. If you feel worse, decrease the amount of time you are exercising.

11. Start moving toward the Paleo diet by removing grains and eating meat and vegetables (see the Fix Your Food chapter).

12. Start working on the *usual suspects* for other causes of physical stress.

13. Start working on any autoimmune issues that may be present.

Action Steps

1. Order the new supplements discussed in this chapter and start the Magnesium Ramp-Up! You can find them under the Constipation Support category in our online store here: us.fullscript.com/welcome/drhirsch

2. Add your new supplements to your Treatment Schedule

3. Track your constipation symptoms on the Symptom Calendar

4. Set alarms on your phone to remind you to take your supplements and to exercise/move, drink your water and squat on the toilet daily.

5. Questions? Ask people in the Facebook group (fb.com/groups/fixyourfatigue) questions like these:

    a. *What was the best treatment for your constipation?*

    b. *Who loves the squatty potty?!*

6. Continue to implement the lifestyle changes and previous treatments you have made so far.

7. Continue eating more meat and vegetables and avoiding grains and sugars.

8. Learn more about the Paleo diet from the handout by Valerie Burke, MSN, in the member area.

9. Congratulations on completing another chapter!

10. Get excited to Fix Your Mold in the next chapter!

Chapter 15:
Fix Your Mold

A my had chronic fatigue for ten years and still wasn't better. She had been treated for heavy metals, Lyme disease, and adrenal fatigue. Those issues had improved on paper, but she still felt awful from the fatigue, brain fog, sinus congestion, chemical sensitivity, and numbness in her hands. When she came to see me, I asked if she ever lived or worked in a place that had water damage or visible mold. "An indoor plumbing leak, a roof leak, a barn, or a flood?" I asked. Amy had grown up in a home that flooded every year. "The basement smelled musty all the time," she said. "I didn't like going down in there." Mold and mycotoxins (mold toxins) were in her body, preventing her from getting better.

Background

It is easier for us to understand things we can see and touch. This is why surgery makes sense to most people. You see a problem, and you manually fix it or cut it out. Things that we can see with fancy laboratory equipment help us make the leap to those things that are too small for us to see with the naked eye. Laboratory tests help us to understand chemical changes and infections occurring in our bodies that we cannot see.

Unfortunately, mold is not something that's easy to see or test for, making it hard to comprehend for both practitioners and patients. Patients will ask me, "If I can't see it in my house, why would it be in my body?" And, "if I had exposure twenty years ago, shouldn't it be out of my body by now?" It doesn't make sense to people that mold and its toxins could be hiding in their bodies for many years, or that it might be in their homes if they don't see it or smell it.

Having mold in your home is also very confusing. It's very common, and lots of people have it in their home, so it's probably not bad, right? If it were a health problem, there would be more education about it, right? Unfortunately, it's a serious public health issue, but because treatment is challenging and testing is confusing, it's easier to just ignore the mold and proceed with life.

According to mold expert Ritchie Shoemaker, MD, fifty percent of all buildings in the United States have water damage, and most of those have mold contamination. It is a significant problem that is becoming more widely accepted and understood.

If you have fatigue, mold toxicity (or mold illness) is one of the most important things to rule out. This is because it is incredibly hard to find a resolution to your fatigue, even if all the other causes are addressed, if mold toxicity is present.

Mold is a fungus that produces mold spores and potent mycotoxins (mold toxins). Current and past exposures to these toxins create problems in the body. Mold will "highjack" the immune system and its ability to prevent infections from causing problems in the body. Consequently, sometimes simply eradicating mold can make other issues resolve themselves. In fact, one small study found that resolving mold toxicity also resolved Lyme disease!

Mold loves to grow in buildings after water damage. Mold feeds on the building materials we use in this country—cellulose, particleboard, dry wall, etc. Mold takes up residence without our knowledge, finding damp, dark recesses in which to hide and thrive. Once it takes hold, it's often quite hard to get rid of. All it takes is one flood or a single leak, such as a leaky plumbing pipe or roof.

Some people think they won't have mold in a new home, but unfortunately, this is not true. To save money on temperature control, newer homes are sealed tightly and do not have good airflow. Poor airflow encourages mold to grow. Further, homes may be exposed to rainfall during construction. The rain moistens the building material and starts growing mold.

Some people are extraordinarily sensitive to mold. In these individuals, mold antigens (allergens) cause the immune system to be constantly attacking the mold, leading to a perpetual state of inflammation and a broad array of symptoms. The following list gives you an idea of just how varied these symptoms may be. The asterisk (*) indicates symptoms that are the *most* strongly suspicious for mold toxicity. Which symptoms do you have?

Symptoms

- Chronic fatigue*

- Muscle weakness

- Muscle cramps

- Joint pain and stiffness

- Sinus*: Postnasal drip, nosebleeds, sinus congestion, chronic sinusitis

- Chronic cough

- Headaches, including migraines

- Ear: Tinnitus, itchy ears*, ear drainage, hearing loss

- Eyes: Red eyes, blurred vision, excess tearing, light sensitivity

- Snoring

- Shortness of breath

- Skin sensitivity

- Gastroesophageal reflux

- Gastrointestinal: Bloating, irritable bowel, diarrhea, gastroparesis (lack of gut peristalsis or movement of food)

- Urinary: Pain with urination, increased urination, excessive thirst

- Vaginal discharge or heavy vaginal bleeding

- Miscarriages

- Vaginal yeast infections*

- Appetite swings

- Sweats, temperature dysregulation

- Hoarseness

- Neurologic*: dizziness, disorientation, tremors, paralysis, numbness, tingling, speech problems, seizures, stroke

- Mood swings*, problems with attention, learning, and memory

- Vertigo

- Metallic taste

- Abdominal pain

- Mold sensitivity (reacting negatively to moldy places)*

- The ability to smell mold upon entering a space*

- High blood pressure

Testing

If you have any of the above symptoms and a history suggestive of mold exposure, get your body and your home tested for mold and mycotoxins.

Your priority is to determine whether you are *currently* being exposed.

To test your home or office for mold, I recommend the following approaches:

- **ERMI Test (Environmental Relative Moldiness Index):** The ERMI test is one of the best tests for measuring mold because it measures the mycotoxin load in your home. This test is especially helpful after remediation because there may still be mycotoxins present even if all of the mold spores have been removed. It costs around $300, and you can find it at mycometrics.com. I used to use mold plates, but I found their results to be inaccurate.

- **Go on vacation:** If you're able to leave your home, your clothes, your car, and your work, do it. If your mold symptoms improve after five days or so, there's probably mold in one of those environments.

- **Professional mold service or a building biologist:** After you have a positive ERMI test, I recommend you hire a building biologist (http://hbelc.org/) to locate the mold and determine how to manage the remediation. These professionals collect air samples and moisture readings. If your home is sick with mold, the next step is remediation. Most building biologists will be able to guide you through this process. In the Pacific Northwest, we use Jason Kester at kesterclear.com.

To see if you have mold in your body, there are two tests I recommend:

- **Urine mycotoxin testing:** checks for mycotoxins in the urine. Mycotoxins are organic poisons produced by molds and fungi. They are secondary metabolites, many known to attach to mitochondrial DNA, and cause damage to nerve cells, the brain, and other organs. Many mycotoxins have been classified as carcinogenic. Unfortunately, you can get rid of mold and still have mycotoxins present in your body and your home. I recommend testing through Real Time Laboratories (your first test is $700 and repeat is $200). You can order it through DirectLabs.com as *Mycotoxin Panel, Total-RTL Kit.*

- **Visual Contrast Test:** The Visual Contrast Test is a test that can be done on your computer screen for $10 to $15. By looking at the contrast in colors, it measures the health of your visual cortex (the vision part of the brain) and whether it has been affected by biotoxin illness. Biotoxin illness includes Lyme disease, so it is not solely a mold test, but it can be very helpful in providing more data. If you do not have Lyme disease, it is a more accurate test for mold toxicity. It is 92% sensitive (meaning that when it is reported that you have biotoxin illness, it is very likely to be true). I recommend repeating this test every three months. It's a great barometer for your treatment progress. When you get into the normal range, you can stop treating mold. You can find the test at VCStest.com or SurvivingMold.com.

To determine if you have mold in your sinuses, consider the MARCoNS test discussed in the Fix Your Sinus Infections chapter. This test is not perfect, however, so if your symptoms are strongly linked to mold exposure, I would still treat the sinuses for mold.

Blood tests also may be used to assess biotoxin illness, but I don't use them. You can learn more about them at SurvivingMold.com.

Step One: Separating From the Mold

Once you find mold in your home, you first must remove the exposure. I cannot emphasize this enough. *You cannot get better if you are still being exposed to mold.*

You have two options:

    a.   Remove yourself from the house (ideal)

b. Remove the mold from your house (not ideal, but more realistic if moving is not possible)

Removing Yourself from the House

If you find out that you are currently being exposed to mold, you and your family should immediately leave the house to allow your health to improve. This is a major step and one that I realize may cause you a lot of anxiety. I totally understand, and I wouldn't make this statement if I didn't think it was absolutely necessary. Unfortunately, I have seen too many cases of people not getting better until they leave their toxic home.

The challenges of moving out of your home are not only financial (and emotional!), but also logistical. What should you take with you? Where should you go? Should you buy or rent? It requires a lot of brainpower to get all of these things in order, which isn't easy if you already have brain fog from mold! This is where a family or community member can be of assistance during this transition.

Here is a list of the different options I have seen patients do:

1. Move in with a family member

2. Move into a studio on a family member's property

3. Build a tiny home on their property

4. Move into a rental

In short, I recommend that you move in with a family member or friend (as soon as possible!) and *leave everything you own* in the house. Then you can figure out how to remediate it as your health improves. First, test the home of your friend/family member (or wherever you move to) to make sure it is safe for you.

Do not commit to another home until you are sure it does not have mold in it! Unfortunately, I have seen people move from one moldy home to another!

What to Take with You

If you're living in a moldy home, you have mold spores and mycotoxins you cannot see covering your clothing and furniture. They travel with you in your car as you transport them to school, work, and everywhere else you go. Leaving one's home is understandably a very difficult thing, but for those who are sick with mold illness, leaving clothes, furniture, and the car behind can mean the difference between getting a little bit better and *the complete resolution of your symptoms.*

Removing Mold from Your Home

If you're unable to leave your home, you need to use air filters to decrease the mold you are breathing. Wear a HEPA mask in the areas that are most toxic (I recommend 3M masks) and place air filters throughout the home. Mold spores are 0.3-microns in size, and the mycotoxins are much smaller at 0.003 microns. The air filter I recommend for mold is the IQAir filter (IQair.com, use code IQ49132 for 10% off). It traps particles down to 0.003, capturing mold spores and mycotoxins.

While you are working on hiring someone to remediate your home, I recommend you start cleaning it yourself with diluted borax (you can find the recipe in the member area) or EC3 products by Sinusitis Wellness (SinusitisWellness.com). *Never use bleach—it will release and spread mold spores.*

Why Husbands Don't Believe Their Wives When It Comes to Mold

It can be quite contentious if family members aren't on the same page when it comes to mold toxicity. Generally, the wife is experiencing symptoms and wants to move or remediate, but the husband does not. The husband usually is not experiencing any symptoms or doesn't have the awareness to notice that he is not well either. Certain genes predispose females to mold illness more often than males. Husbands need to trust their wives. Their symptoms are real, mold illness is a real problem, and you need to support each other through this process.

Treatment

Once you have removed yourself from the source of exposure, you can begin to clean out your body and restore your immune system. To do this, I use my five-step Fix Your Mold plan:

1. Flush the mold out of its hiding places (with biofilm disruptors)

2. Bind it up (with binding agents)

3. Destroy it (with antifungals)

4. Starve it (with an antifungal diet)

5. Move it out of the body through the detoxification pathways (with detoxifiers)

Step 1: Biofilm Disruptors

Molds living in biofilms tend to be impervious to antifungal treatments without the addition of an agent to break up these films. Biofilm is a collagenous material deposited on mucous membranes that allows these fungi to hide and swap their DNA with other infections. Biofilm disruptors are usually enzymes that break up biofilm. These enzymes not only break up the biofilms for mold, but also for any other infections that may be cohabitating.

Step 2: Binding Agents

Next, binding agents capture the mold and mycotoxins so that they can be eliminated from the body. I have found that taking activated charcoal twice daily is usually treatment enough, but I have used zeolites, modified citrus pectin, and prescription bile sequestering agents like cholestyramine as well. I believe cholestyramine to be the strongest treatment available, however, it is very poorly tolerated by patients, so I no longer use it.

Step 3: Antifungals

Mold is a fungus. Like yeast, it can be killed with antifungals. Signs of fungus in the body include itching (on the skin and in the ears and anus), skin rashes, vaginal yeast infections, feeling worse after eating sugar (and grains), and toenail fungus. I have used natural (herbal) antifungals for many years, but have found that on many occasions prescription antifungals were needed. I've had the most success using prescription oral fluconazole (Diflucan) and nystatin. Always use Daily Liver Formula (by Gaia) with Diflucan to prevent liver damage. Mold loves to live in the sinuses. Allergic fungal sinusitis (AFS) was found to account for the vast majority of cases of chronic sinusitis—a whopping 96 percent—by a Mayo Clinic study.

If you have symptoms of chronic sinusitis like post-nasal drip, sinus infections, and sinus congestion, I will use antifungals sprays into the nose like amphotericin B and itraconazole, as well as sinus ozone treatments.

Ozone is not the toxic ozone in the atmosphere, but a lower dose activated oxygen therapy that is wonderfully anti-microbial (bug killer). We use it in several different ways in our clinic with great results. You can learn more here: DrsOzone.com.

Step 4: Antifungal Diet

The antifungal diet is challenging, but it must be done. Molds feed on sugars, vinegar (fermented products), and other fungi. This includes fruits, grains, potatoes, sweeteners, soda pop, mushrooms, kombucha, Cole slaw, sauerkraut, pickles, cheese, peanuts, and coffee (both high in molds). My antifungal diet handout explains what you can eat, meal plans, a shopping list, and snack ideas. You can download it from the member area (fixyourfatigue.org/members).

Step 5: Detoxification Support

Our bodies gather toxins in our lymph system, then move them through different phases in the liver and into the kidneys and intestines. Eventually, these toxins will be excreted out our stool, urine, breath, and skin. Consequently, my favorite detox protocols involve therapies that facilitate these processes. I recommend a combination of herbs, infrared saunas, oxygen and ozone therapy, massage therapy, exercise, IV multivitamins (Myers' "cocktails"), magnesium, and glutathione, the body's main antioxidant and detoxifier.

Total Body Load

Many fatigue patients come in with multiple infections and toxins, and their immune system is on complete overload. This combination of the *usual suspects* – heavy metals, chemicals, molds, infections, allergies, EMFs, and emotions – is your total body load (or total body burden). This load must be lightened before the immune system can function properly.

If you have multiple issues, such as Lyme disease and its many co-infections, the treatment protocol can be extensive. But you may not need to do ALL of it—just key parts. In many cases, you knock out one major offender, and the rest fall like dominos. The protocols I'm presenting in this book have an advantage in that they have multiple therapeutic pathways that work together to facilitate your healing as quickly and efficiently as possible.

Now that you understand how significant mold can be, please start immediately to clear your home and your body. The sooner you start this protocol, the sooner you will reduce your suffering and get your life back!

Summary

If you have fatigue, mold is one of the most important things to get rid of, but it can also be one of the most challenging. Because of the potent mycotoxins it produces, mold can create problems in the body from current and past exposures. Sometimes merely eradicating mold from the body can make other issues fall like dominos, so it's important to address it from the get-go. Some individuals are especially sensitive to mold as a result of their particular genetic makeup.

Because it affects so many systems in the body, mold can produce a broad array of symptoms, from fatigue to gastrointestinal symptoms to neurological abnormalities and autoimmune disease. Mold also likes to hide out in the sinuses and is particularly fond of creating biofilms.

Both patients and their homes should be tested for mold to rule out ongoing sources of exposure. It is imperative for patients to take the challenging step of removing themselves and their families from a moldy home. In addition to receiving treatment for mold illness, remediation of the home will be necessary.

The protocol pushes mold out of its hiding places in the body with biofilm disruptors, kills it with antifungals, binds it with charcoal, and supports the body's detoxification pathways with herbs, vitamins, and minerals.

The Plan

Once you determine that you have mold in your body that is affecting your health, I recommend that you begin treatment.

1. Start Interfase Plus 2 caps two times per day in between meals to disrupt the biofilm. If you have a sensitivity to eggs, use Natto-Serrizime 2 caps two times per day in between meals instead.

2. Start Activated Charcoal 6 caps two times per day to bind up the mold. Take it ninety minutes away from all food and supplements. Recommended times are at 10 a.m. and before bed. If you can only do once a day, then take 10-12 caps before bed. Take all other evening supplements 90 minutes before this.

3. Start Phytostan 2 caps three times per day for an herbal antifungal treatment.

4. Start Yeast Formula 2 caps three times per day for an herbal antifungal treatment.

If the herbal formulas are not strong enough after three months, then have your provider prescribe the following:

5. Diflucan 200 mg per day for three months minimum

6. Nystatin 1 million units three times per day for three months minimum

7. Since Diflucan can damage the liver, you'll need to take Daily Liver Formula 2 per day every time you take the Diflucan.

8. Start the antifungal diet for a minimum of three months. Exclude fruits, grains, potatoes, sweeteners, soda pop, mushrooms, kombucha, Cole slaw, sauerkraut, pickles, cheese, peanuts, and coffee. Download the handout for more information on the specifics.

Once your fungal symptoms are completely resolved for at least two months, you can stop the antifungals and the antifungal diet. These symptoms include itchy skin, itchy anus, itchy ears, vaginal yeast infections, skin rashes, and toenail fungus. If you don't have any of these symptoms, then stop after three months.

9. Start ACG glutathione 1 spray two times per day and increase every week by 1 spray two times per day up to 12 sprays two times per day.

10. Start far infrared saunas three times per week. Start at ten minutes per treatment (five minutes if you are chemically sensitive and react strongly to treatments) and increase by one minute each week until you are up to thirty to forty-five minutes per treatment. If you

feel worse afterward, then decrease your minutes and advance more slowly. Far infrared saunas remove toxins from the body's tissues at the cellular level, so you are detoxifying before you even sweat! I recommend low EMF saunas from HeavenlyHeatSaunas.com and Sunlighten.com.

11. If you have nutrient deficiencies of B12, folate, and magnesium, make sure they are replaced to support detoxification and take a good multivitamin like Innate One Daily.

12. If you have access to IV therapy:

    a. Start IV "Myers Cocktail," alternating every 48 hours with IV glutathione. The "Myers Cocktail" is an intravenous formula containing vitamins and minerals (B vitamins, vitamin C, calcium, and magnesium) to boost methylation (phase two detoxification of the liver).

    b. Start IV glutathione 300 milligrams. Increase by 300 milligrams every other dose up to 1800 milligrams.

For sinus symptoms related to mold, I recommend the following:

1. Start Amphotericin B nasal spray (compounded prescription from your provider), twice a day for two months for sinus fungus only (ineffective against bacteria).

2. Start ACS 200 Extra Strength Nasal Spray (by Results RNA) 2 sprays two times per day. This is a colloidal silver spray effective against both fungi and bacteria

3. Start sinus ozone two to three times per week for ten to thirty treatments. Find someone in your area at DrsOzone.com or purchase your own system at TrulyHeal.

Important Treatment Notes

If you are no longer in a moldy environment, treatment is usually needed for six to twelve months or until your urine mycotoxins level reaches zero or your VCS test is in the normal range. Research has shown that if you stop before this time, symptoms will return. While you usually will see symptom improvement in the first few months, it is important to continue for this duration. You will also be combining treatments from other causes as you go through this process.

Action Steps

1. Order the new supplements discussed in this chapter. You can find them under the Mold Support category in our online store here: us.fullscript.com/welcome/drhirsch

2. Add your new supplements to your Treatment Schedule

3. Track your symptoms on the Symptom Calendar

4. Set alarms on your phone to remind you to take your supplements

5. Download the Antifungal Diet from the member area at fixyourfatigue.org/members.

6. Questions? Ask people in the Facebook group questions like these:

    a. *What mold symptoms do you have?*

    b. *Which is better to use to clean the house: borax or EC3 products?*

    c. *Anyone know a good building biologist in my area?*

7. Continue to implement the lifestyle changes you have made and the previous treatments.

8. Congratulations on completing another chapter!

9. Get ready to Fix Your Heavy Metals and Chemicals next!

Chapter 16:
Fix Your Heavy Metal and Chemical Toxicity

My shoulders ached. My neck hurt. I had body pain all day long. It wasn't until I tested and treated myself for mercury toxicity that my body pain went away and my fatigue improved significantly from a 5/10 to 7/10.

Background

Heavy metal and chemical toxicity was one of the most significant factors in my fatigue. As a child, I loved tuna fish sandwiches. I ate them daily for lunch. Unfortunately, I didn't know that tens of thousands of pounds of mercury were being dumped into our oceans every year by coal plants or that my amalgam fillings were releasing mercury into my body. Add in a history of exposure to plastics, contact with formaldehyde from gross anatomy class in medical school, chronic constipation, and a genetic detoxification problem (MTHFR), and I had a perfect storm of toxicity and dysfunction.

Besides causing chronic fatigue, toxicity from heavy metals and chemicals has also been implicated as causes of neuropathy, inflammation, fibromyalgia, cardiovascular disease, and autoimmunity. Thanks to today's modern industrial, agricultural, medical, cosmetic, and technological practices, we are unknowingly exposed to heavy metals and toxic chemicals on a daily basis. Our physiology is poorly equipped to rid our bodies of these foreign agents, and they accumulate over time in our tissues. Eventually, they cause dysfunction and disease.

The question is not whether your body has been exposed to heavy metal and chemical contamination, *but rather how much and what kind*. These toxic agents are ubiquitous, and some level of exposure is simply unavoidable. A growing number of studies are finding that hundreds of toxic chemicals are detectable in babies' bodies before they're even born. In one study, cord blood from babies and breast milk each contained more than two hundred different toxic chemicals.

Consequently, our plan is going to include removing toxins from your body and avoiding new exposures.

The following list illustrates some common sources of exposure, *but there are many more*, far too many to include. Just from this sampling, you can appreciate how ubiquitous heavy metals and chemicals are in the world today. Collectively they can wreak havoc on your health. Some of these contaminants are no longer in use, but they are still found in our bodies from previous exposures and from those we acquired in the womb from our mothers.

Heavy Metals:

- **Mercury**: fish and seafood, dental fillings (amalgam), pharmaceuticals, fluorescent light bulbs, paints, and art supplies

- **Lead**: Paint, batteries, cigarette smoke, canned food, ceramics, old pipes, solders, PVC, gasoline, auto exhaust, art supplies and other pigments

- **Aluminum**: Aluminum cookware and coffee pots, deodorants, baby formula, cosmetics, refined flour, antacids and other drugs

- **Cadmium**: Black rubber, burned motor oil, secondhand smoke, ceramics, evaporated milk, fertilizers, fungicides, soft drinks

- **Arsenic**: Wood treatments, herbicides, pesticides, semiconductors, paints and dyes, soaps, rice, commercial juices

- **Nickel**: Cigarettes, cookware, diesel exhaust, foods, batteries, jewelry, dental materials, prostheses, welding materials

- **Barium**: Medical imaging, paint, decorative glass, insecticides, peanuts

- **Tin**: Foods, water pipes, rubber, solders, dyes, pigments, bleaching agents, rodent poisons, insecticides, fungicides

Chemicals:

- **Fire Retardants (PBDEs):** Clothing, furniture, baby carriers, car seats, strollers, cribs, nursing pillows, baby blankets

- **Bisphenol A, phthalates**: Plastic water bottles and baby bottles, canned foods, dental sealants, and thousands of other products

- **Perfluorochemicals (PFCs):** Nonstick cookware, stain-resistant carpets, furniture, fabrics, fish

- **Dioxins**: Meat, poultry, dairy, fish, PVC, bleaching agents, bleached coffee filters, tampons, and paper products, especially bleached varieties

- **Pesticides**: Glyphosate (Round-Up), DDT, polychlorinated biphenyls (PCBs), dioxin, heptachlor, chlordane, Aldrin, and Dieldrin

Symptoms

Acute heavy metal and chemical toxicity (toxicity that has occurred over a short period of time) has different symptoms than that of chronic (long-term) exposure. Symptoms of acute toxicity include:

- Nausea

- Vomiting

- Sweating

- Headache

- Difficulty breathing

- Impaired cognitive, motor, and language skills

- Sudden, severe cramping and/or convulsions

- Symptoms of chronic heavy metal and chemical toxicity include:

  - Chronic fatigue

  - Neuropathy (numbness and tingling)

  - Muscle pain

  - Joint pain

- Digestive distress and reduced ability to properly assimilate and utilize fats

- Brain fog

- Memory loss

- Anosmia (loss of smell)

- Depression

- Impaired blood sugar regulation

- Female reproductive problems such as menstrual difficulties, infertility, miscarriage, pre-eclampsia, pregnancy-induced hypertension (high blood pressure), and premature birth

Testing for Heavy Metals and Chemicals

Assessing your exposure to heavy metals and chemicals involves your health history and laboratory testing.

I recommend testing for heavy metal toxicity using a pre- and post-urine challenge (or provocation) test through Doctors Data Laboratory (DirectLabs.com). Most heavy metals are bound up in tissues, so we stimulate or "provoke" their release using a chelation agent, usually Succimer (Dimercaptosuccinic acid, also known as DMSA), which is FDA-approved for the treatment of lead poisoning. The term "chelate" is Latin for *claw*—these agents grab (bind) the heavy metals in tissues, pulling them out into the bloodstream where they can be eliminated (and measured) in the urine.

Testing for chemicals toxicity is also done with a urine test. I recommend the Toxic CORE by Genova Diagnostics

(DirectLabs.com). It looks at the chemical deposition in fat cells and is relatively accurate, but unfortunately, quite expensive at $700.

If you do not have access to laboratory testing, that's okay. Unless you are living "off the grid" without electricity or the conveniences of modern living, you've probably had significant heavy metal and chemical exposure, and you can proceed with the gentle heavy metal and chemical removal protocol I will discuss.

You can also test your water for heavy metals like lead. I recommend contacting Doctors Data Laboratories at 800-323-2784 for a test kit. The cost is around $150.

Treatment

Reversing disease requires reducing the body's total toxic burden of heavy metals and chemicals. This reduction allows the immune system, the detoxification systems, and all of the body's systems to function more efficiently.

Treatment includes:

1. Opening up the body's detoxification pathways

2. Removing the heavy metals and chemicals from the body

3. Making lifestyle choices that minimize further accumulation of heavy metals and chemical toxicity

4. Depending on the amount of heavy metals present, your severity of symptoms, and where you are in the process, I will use different treatments.

Natural Treatments

As always, I like to start with natural treatments as long as they work.

To open up the body's detoxification pathways, I use vitamin B12, folate, alpha lipoic acid, magnesium, n-acetylcysteine, glutathione, uva ursi, and marshmallow extract. I will also consider additional liver support with herbs like milk thistle, dandelion, burdock, and stinging nettle.

- **Glutathione** is one of the most powerful antioxidants, known for its ability to protect the body against the damages caused by heavy metal toxicity and environmental toxins. It is the predominant antioxidant found in the liver and breaks down wastes, toxins, and heavy metals into less harmful compounds.

- **N-Acetyl-Cysteine (NAC)** is a precursor to glutathione and has powerful antioxidant and liver-protective actions. In addition to protecting the body from oxidative damage, NAC can be used for heavy metal damage, and where there is a need, to rebuild the liver and promote optimal detoxification. Research also shows that NAC can be used as a provoking agent for mercury.

- **Alpha Lipoic Acid** (ALA) is a broad-spectrum antioxidant that acts as an orally active recycler of glutathione. It is believed that ALA participates in the chelation process because it can easily penetrate cell membranes. It binds with circulating heavy metals to prevent them from causing cellular damage.

To bind up and remove heavy metals from the body, some natural treatments include modified citrus pectin, chlorella, garlic, cilantro, zeolites, and saunas.

- **Chlorella (*Chlorella regularis*)** is a green alga considered to be one of the most nutrient-dense substances on earth. It has been shown to support the healthy function of the digestive, circulatory, and pulmonary systems. Its role in heavy metal chelation has been extensively researched. Findings show it can bind with metals such as mercury, lead, and cadmium. As with alginates, chlorella also plays an integral role in helping to prevent the reabsorption of minerals after they have been released from the tissues.

- **Garlic (*Allium sativum*)** is one of the richest dietary sources of various health-promoting sulfur compounds. These components help to oxidize heavy metals, allowing for their excretion. Garlic also protects blood cells from the damage caused by metals that appear in the bloodstream as they work their way through the detoxification process. Garlic can also stimulate the production of glutathione.

- **Cilantro (*Coriandrum sativum*)** is a botanical capable of mobilizing mercury, cadmium, lead, and aluminum in the central nervous system.

- **Zeolites** have open, cage-like structures or "frameworks" that facilitate the capture and containment of other molecules. They bind very specifically to heavy metals by three different mechanisms: the charge of the molecule, the size of the molecule, and the binding coefficient. A binding coefficient is a measure of the attraction between a molecule and its mate. The binding coefficient between zeolite and heavy metals is very high, ensuring that the metals are more likely to stay bound to zeolite than to anything else, reducing the odds of reabsorption.

ACZ Nano is my favorite zeolite product because it's a nanoparticle, which means it doesn't go through the gut. When sprayed into your mouth, it is quickly absorbed through your mucus membranes to reach your cells and organs. It binds to heavy metals, chemicals, radiation, and a little bit to mold, so it's a wonderful catch-all for many of the toxins with which we regularly come into contact.

- **Saunas** are the best way to remove chemicals from the body, especially far infrared saunas. We can detoxify through the skin through sweating. Far infrared saunas detoxify the body from the inside out, by heating the tissues several inches deep to cause a rise in core body temperature. This stimulates the circulatory system to increase oxygen through the body and enhances the metabolic processes. Consequently, even before you sweat, you are detoxifying. This is especially important for patients who have difficulty sweating or do not sweat on a regular basis. Repeated use of the sauna slowly restores circulation and the ability for toxins to move from the cellular level to the skin's surface. The toxins are then removed by sweating. The heat and the wavelength generated by far infrared saunas also can kill off viruses and other microorganisms.

Pharmaceutical Treatment

If I need a more aggressive approach because the natural treatment isn't working as fast as I would like, I will use DMSA orally. Dosing is typically 100-500 mg three times per day, on for three days and off for eleven days, for a minimum of eight cycles or four months.

Side Effects of Chelation

When you are chelating (binding up) heavy metals, the goal is to bind them up and excrete them out of the body. Unfortunately, it's not a perfect process, and chelated heavy metals can sometimes be re-deposited into other tissues before they are excreted out of the body. This essentially re-exposes you to the toxins and can result in worsening symptoms.

If I am concerned about this process in a patient, I get around this by performing a slow detox with gentle chelators over one and a half to two years. This decreases the chances of heavy metal re-deposition. People see improvement in their symptoms in the first few months, but I find safety in the long game where slow and steady wins the race.

Another concern is mineral depletion. Often, chelation agents can bind to minerals indiscriminately, so you end up removing minerals from the body along with the heavy metals. This can cause mineral deficiencies. The risk is much lower with zeolites because they are so specific to the molecules you want to remove from your body. However, during heavy metal chelation, I recommend a good multivitamin and multi-mineral complex.

Additionally, heavy metals and chemicals exacerbate chronic infections. They suppress the immune system, create biofilms (the hiding place for infections), and damage mitochondria, allowing infections to propagate. When you start removing these toxins, the biofilm becomes disrupted and releases infections. Your immune system becomes stronger and can more easily resolve chronic infections. Be aware that releasing metals can put bugs on the move, which may increase your symptoms and make infections more apparent. See the Fix Your Stealth Infections chapter for more information.

Reducing Your Heavy Metal and Chemical Exposure

Removing heavy metals and chemicals from your body will decrease your total body burden and improve your symptoms. Once you have done this, the next step is to remove the ongoing daily exposures that made you sick in the first place!

Please note: this step is optional! It can get very overwhelming and expensive adhering to all of the steps I recommend below, and they don't need to happen right now. Many of my patients wait until their fatigue has resolved or their energy is above a 7/10 before they make some of these environmental changes.

Toxins are everywhere. They are found in our water, food, cosmetics, cars, and air (name a few). Here is how to remove these exposures:

1. To avoid pesticides in food, I recommend consuming as much organic food as possible. When it is not possible, consume organic foods that are on the Dirty Dozen list (these foods are laden with pesticides) and non-organic foods that are on the Clean Fifteen list (foods that do not have lots of pesticides). I have included these lists from Environmental Working Group in the member area of my website.

2. Avoid mercury in fish. Unfortunately, an enormous amount of mercury is generated during coal production and ends up in our oceans. Since mercury is stored in fat, the bigger the fish, the more mercury it has. Consequently, I recommend limiting your fish

intake to the smaller fish like anchovies and sardines. My wife, Stacy, makes a great sardine salad (it tastes like tuna fish salad) that I will share with you in the member area. I consume most of my fish oil through supplements that have undergone third-party testing to ensure they are free of heavy metals.

3. For pollutants in the air, I recommend Austin Air filters (AustinAir.com) for general air filtration and IQair filters (IQair.com, use code IQ49132 for 10% off) for air that has mold and mold toxins in it.

4. For toxins in your water, I recommend Aquasana (Aquasana.com) for whole house carbon water filtration or countertop water filters. I highly recommend taking baths and showers without chlorine – a benefit of the whole house filter.

5. For toxins in cosmetics, I recommend that patients stop wearing any product with fragrance. This includes perfume/cologne, shampoo, skin lotion, and scented candles. These are all usually toxic. I then recommend that they assess the toxicity of their cosmetics at ewg.org/skindeep. This is a great website that has tested most of the cosmetics on the market and will tell you how toxic your cosmetics are. If they are toxic, you can choose less toxic options.

6. To reduce toxin exposure while in your car, I recommend that you always drive with "recycled air" on. Additionally, I recommend a car air filter by E.L Foust (Auto/RV Air Purifier at foustco.com) if you feel worse in your car or if you have a long commute.

7. You simply can't avoid all of these toxins, so supporting the body's detoxification pathways by eating a clean diet and following these strategies is an

extremely important part of getting well and living in today's toxic world.

Summary

A high body burden of heavy metals and chemicals may be a significant factor in your fatigue. Our bodies are poorly equipped to rid themselves of heavy metals and chemicals, and they are very prevalent in today's environment. Notable toxins include the heavy metals mercury, aluminum, and lead, as well as chemicals like dioxins, PBDEs, glyphosate, and BPA.

Urine challenge tests with provocation are useful in assessing heavy metal and chemical toxicity. Levels taken before and after provocation allow you to estimate how many heavy metals are locked up in the tissues of the body. Treatment involves using herbs, zeolites, and sometimes DMSA to help pull toxic compounds out of tissues, and glutathione to open up detoxification pathways.

The Plan

Our plan consists of opening detoxification pathways, binding up the heavy metals and chemicals, and removing them from the body.

This plan is a gentle removal of heavy metals and chemicals that is done slowly over one to two years.

1. Start ACG Glutathione 1 spray two times per day. Increase weekly by 1 spray two times per day up to 12 sprays two times per day. Take for two years. This opens up detoxification pathways and is the body's main antioxidant.

2. Start Alpha Lipoic Acid 1 cap two times per day. Take for two years. This is a natural chelator and recycles glutathione. It also supports the kidneys and liver in detoxification and heals mitochondria.

3. Start Magnesium Chelate 1 tab per night and increase every three nights by 1 tab until you get soft stools per the Magnesium Ramp-Up. This supports detoxification and excretion pathways.

4. Start using a far infrared sauna (if available) five minutes per day and increase by one minute every week up to thirty to forty-five minutes per day. If you feel worse afterward, decrease the time you are spending in the sauna and the frequency. Consider purchasing a low EMF sauna from HeavenlyHeatSaunas.com or Sunlighten.com.

5. In one month, start Metal-X-Synergy 3 caps per night before bed two hours away from all medications and supplements to avoid binding those up. Increase to 6 caps in one month. This is a combination of cilantro, chlorella, modified citrus pectin, garlic, alpha lipoic acid, and glutathione to bind and remove heavy metals.

6. In one month, also start Heavy Metal Support 2 capsules at dinner and 2 caps before bed every day. This contains minerals to prevent mineral depletion from chelation, supports detoxification pathways and protects the liver and kidneys. It contains l-methionine, uva ursi, alpha lipoic acid and marshmallow extract. Additional vitamin B12 and folate may be needed based on your test results (please see the Fix Your Nutrients chapter).

7. In two months, start ACZ Nano 1 spray two times per day. Increase weekly by 1 spray two times per day up to 10 sprays two times per day. Take for two years. This binds up heavy metals and chemicals.

8. Start removing daily exposures if it's not too overwhelming for you, by going to ewg.org/skindeep to determine if your cosmetics are making you sick.

If you have elevated levels of heavy metals on your urine testing, consider the more aggressive protocol:

1. Start #1-4 above to open up detoxification pathways.

2. In one month, start DMSA 500mg three times per day, three days on and eleven days off. Continue for four months. This will replace #5 and #7 above.

3. In one month, start Heavy Metal Support 2 capsules at dinner and 2 caps before bed every day.

4. Start removing daily exposures if it's not too overwhelming for you, by going to ewg.org/skindeep to determine if your cosmetics are making you sick.

Action Steps

1. Order the new supplements discussed in this chapter. You can find them under the Heavy Metal & Chemical Support category in our online store here: us.fullscript.com/welcome/drhirsch

2. Add your new supplements to your Treatment Schedule

3. Set alarms on your phone to remind you to take your supplements

4. Download the EWG Dirty Dozen and Clean Fifteen lists from the member area at fixyourfatigue.org/members.

5. Download the Sardine Salad recipe from the member area.

6. Questions? Ask people in the Facebook group (fb.com/groups/fixyourfatigue) questions like these:

    a. *Who else found out how much lead their lipstick has?*

    b. *Which of your cosmetics had the most toxins in it?*

    c. *Anyone have any other good recipes that include sardines?*

7. Continue to implement the lifestyle changes you have made and the previous treatments.

8. Congratulations on completing another chapter! You are amazing!

9. Get ready to Fix Your Stealth Infections next!

Chapter 17:
Fix Your Stealth Infections

W*hen Kathy came to see me, she had pain and burning on the bottoms of her feet, sleep problems, anxiety, depression, neck pain, low thyroid, muscle cramps, and headaches. Once we started treating the bacteria Bartonella, all of her symptoms improved.*

Background

I never wanted to treat chronic infections, especially Lyme disease, caused by *Borrelia Burgdorferi*, and its co-infections (also known as *stealth* infections for their ability to hide from the immune system). They seemed to be too challenging to treat, and the treatments were too hard on the body. I wanted to leave these cases to the Lyme-literate medical doctors (called LLMDs). I believed if we made the immune system strong enough and replaced nutrient and hormonal deficiencies everyone would be able to fight off any infection.

Unfortunately, I learned that this wasn't the case. I also learned that there were natural options to treating chronic infections and that treatments could be successful without antibiotics. Once I started treating chronic infections, I was able to resolve and reverse some of the most stubborn medical problems I encountered, including chronic fatigue, eczema, psoriasis, Hashimoto's hypothyroidism, and rheumatoid arthritis.

Friend or Foe?

Most people are surprised to hear that our bodies are made up of 90 percent non-human (bacteria, virus, fungi) cells and 10 percent human cells. It's like we are visitors in our own bodies! The bacteria, viruses, and fungi that inhabit our bodies (called the microbiome or microorganisms) are incredibly important for our overall function, and we were made to live with them in harmony.

When stress is placed on the body by one of the *usual suspects* (heavy metals, chemicals, molds, infections, allergies, EMFs, or emotions), dysfunction occurs, and the immune system can no longer keep the microbiome in balance. This imbalance in the microbiome is called dysbiosis. Consequently, some of the microorganisms take advantage of the environment and proliferate, leading to infection. The immune system will then seek to restore balance by eliminating these infections through a process called inflammation.

Inflammation is a series of messages that targets an area where the infection is present. It recruits the immune system to attack this area. If the immune system is successful, the amount of the infection is reduced to its original form, and balance is restored. If it is not successful, the infection will persist, as will the inflammation. The inflammation notifies the body of the presence of a foreign substance (in this case, an infection) by causing pain and dysfunction at the area of interest. This underlying chronic inflammation is what causes so much of the pain, dysfunction, and symptoms I see in my patients on a daily basis.

Symptoms

Infections can produce fascinating symptoms in different parts of the body. For example, the bacteria *Bartonella*, which Kathy experienced, lives in the blood and presents problems in the muscles, the feet, the thyroid, the neck, the gut and the nervous system.

Stealth infections are often found in organs, as well, and can cause almost any kind of symptom, including:

- Insomnia

- Chronic fatigue

- Cognitive dysfunction: brain fog, memory loss

- Urinary symptoms: pain with urination, urination at night, urinary urgency and frequency

- Temperature changes: Cyclical fevers, night or day sweats, cold hands and feet

- Muscle pain: neck pain, headaches, and muscle cramping (especially in calves and feet)

- Joint pain: Migratory and non-migratory, knee, foot, hand, hip, shoulder pain

- Mood issues: depression, anxiety, panic attacks

- Neuropathies: numbness, tingling, and shooting pains

- Hormonal deficiencies: adrenal, thyroid, sex hormones

The Most Common Stealth Infections

These common stealth infections contribute to fatigue:

- **Epstein–Barr virus (EBV)** is a virus responsible for infectious mononucleosis (remember the "kissing disease" you had as a teen?). It commonly causes memory loss, "brain fog," and fatigue.

- **Babesia**, typically spread by ticks, is a malaria-like parasite that can infect red blood cells to cause babesiosis. It typically causes severe sleep problems, cognitive issues, sweating during the day and/or night, feeling hot (but different than a hot flash), suicidal thoughts, and panic attacks.

- **Bartonella** are gram-negative bacteria responsible for "cat scratch disease" and trench fever. They have been associated with a variety of conditions, including hepatitis (liver infection), endocarditis (heart infection), encephalopathy (brain infection), and meningoencephalitis (brain lining infection). *Bartonella* can be spread by ticks, fleas, biting flies, and lice. Symptoms include pain on the bottoms of the feet (often mistaken for plantar fasciitis), stretch marks on the lower back, muscle cramps, abdominal pain, sleep problems, anxiety, depression, diarrhea, cold hands and feet, thyroid dysfunction, heart palpitations, neuropathies, muscle pain (like fibromyalgia), neck pain, headaches, migraines, occasional fevers, Raynaud's syndrome, and joint pain in the hands, thumbs, knees, or hips.

- **Borrelia** or "Lyme" disease is caused by the spirochete bacterium *Borrelia burgdorferi*, typically spread through the bite of a tick, although evidence supports other vectors (including fleas, biting flies, and sexual activity). Often (but not always) it presents initially as a skin rash. Unfortunately, only 10 percent of people with Lyme disease have a rash. *Borrelia* can spread to other tissues, including the brain, joints, heart, peripheral nerves, muscles, and others.

Symptoms may develop immediately or years later, as the organism can remain dormant and take on alternate forms, such as cysts and biofilms. Symptoms include joint pain that moves around the body, neuropathies (numbness and tingling), and mild sleep, mood, and cognitive (brain function) symptoms.

- **Mycoplasma** are the smallest free-living organisms, uniquely lacking cell walls, which makes them resistant to many conventional antibiotics and treatments. At least seventeen species have been identified. They prefer mucosal tissues such as respiratory or urogenital tracts, although they may invade the bloodstream. *Mycoplasma* are a common cause of "walking" pneumonia. Symptoms can be similar to *Borrelia*. *Mycoplasma* are commonly found among those with autoimmune diseases such as rheumatoid arthritis and multiple sclerosis.

Testing

Infections can be identified by the symptoms they cause and by diagnostic testing in blood. Blood testing is controversial. Here are the options for blood testing and the reasons why they are controversial:

- **PCR testing:** This testing looks for the DNA of the infection in the blood. Because many of these infections can cause problems at low levels and can hide in tissues, this test usually does not detect them.

- **Serology testing**: This testing looks at the immune system's response to the infection. Consequently, this test depends on an intact immune system. If someone has any of the *usual suspects* (heavy metals, chemicals, molds, infections, electromagnetic frequencies, allergies, or emotional trauma), their immune system is probably dysfunctional, and this testing is less accurate.

Treating Based On Symptoms

As you can see, our testing is imperfect. In medical school, I was taught that 90 percent of any diagnosis would be made by listening to the patient and asking questions, 5 percent from the physical exam, and 5 percent from laboratory testing. This is absolutely true.

Our bodies tell us when something is wrong; we just have to listen. When we listen to our bodies and convey this information to a knowledgeable medical provider, we can get guidance and get better.

I highly recommend that you become the expert on your body. Observe your body and note all the places where you have pain and dysfunction. Write down that list and bring it to your medical provider so they can help you. The descriptions above indicate how varied and disparate symptoms can be for a particular infection. Did you find your symptoms in any of those infection descriptions?

You might be surprised to know that even the CDC considers Lyme to be a clinical diagnosis! This means that based on the signs and symptoms of the patient, the provider can determine the diagnosis. Yes, that's correct. The CDC uses serology testing for epidemiologic studies and not for diagnosis.

That said, we always want to gather all of the data available to make the best decisions for treatment. We need the patient's history of their symptoms, physical signs of illness, and laboratory findings to come to the best conclusion and decision for treatment.

Treatment: Do This First

In almost every case, patients with chronic fatigue have *multiple infections* at play, so how do you go about treating them? Where do you start?

Once you have determined from testing and symptoms which infections are present, you can begin to treat. However, it is important to emphasize that I've had the most success eliminating infections *when other toxins are treated first (and in conjunction)*. These toxins are (you guessed it) the *usual suspects*!

These *usual suspects* (heavy metals, chemicals, molds, infections, allergies, emotions and electromagnetic frequencies) encourage infection growth in the following ways:

1. They distract the immune system from its normal bug-killing actions

2. They clog up detoxification and elimination pathways, so infections are not easily removed from the body

3. They thicken the blood to make it easier for infections to travel throughout the body

4. They build up biofilms in which infections hide and create superbugs. That's right. These infections will hide in places called biofilms and swap DNA with each other to form superbugs.

Once you have removed the *usual suspects* or started on the path to do so, you will be much more successful at treating any infections that are present. That is why this chapter on infections is placed *after* you have started addressing the rest of the *usual suspects*!

Treatment

When you have multiple infections, the order in which you go after them matters. I've found it most effective first to pursue the infections that create the greatest positive shifts in the body with the fewest side effects. Then, proceed to the "low-hanging fruit," the ones that are easiest to kill. As these infections die and your immune system gets stronger, you will be able to remove some of the more challenging infections like *Borrelia* (Lyme disease) when the time is right. All of these treatments typically require a minimum of six months, but treatments are layered; you will be going after more than one at a time. Consequently, the more infections you need to treat, the longer your treatment time will be.

I go after stealth infections in this general order:

1. *Bartonella*

2. *Babesia*

3. *Epstein-Barr virus*

4. *Mycoplasma*

5. *Anaplasma*

6. *Borrelia*

These clever microbes are masters of stealth and disguise. Our strategy is to force them out of their hiding places (biofilms) and their protective forms (cysts), so they are more susceptible to being killed. We must support the immune system during this process, as it's our number one ally in restoring the microbial balance in the body.

A biofilm is a jelly-like material that allows colonies of bacteria and other infections to hide from the immune system and treatments. In the biofilm, these infections can swap DNA with each other and create superbugs. Biofilm disruptors include enzymes and heavy metal chelators (binders that remove heavy metals from our organs and biofilm).

The simplest, most powerful way of removing these infections is with the infection-specific herbal complexes by Byron White Formulas. These elegant formulas are very powerful herbal combinations; they require the support of a practitioner knowledgeable in how to use them. In fact, you cannot buy them except through an approved practitioner. If you search online for these formulas, you'll find lots of negative reviews. This is because they are so powerful that you must go slow and make sure you have enough detoxification (and die-off) support to handle the treatment. I am going to give you a general approach in *The Plan* section, but there are many nuances with which I recommend you get support. This support might come from a practitioner knowledgeable in these products or continuing education with me.

If you do not have access to Byron White Formulas (unfortunately, I do not have them in my online store yet for you), I recommend the Cowden Support Program. Other treatments that I recommend by infection include:

- **Bartonella**: Neem, Usnea Lichen, Grapefruit seed extract, pokeroot

- **Babesia**: Artemesia, Noni, Cat's Claw (Samento)

- **Epstein-Barr virus**: Monolaurin, Olive Leaf, Reishi, Garlic (Allicin), Thuja

- **Mycoplasma**: Uva Ursi, Usnea Lichen, Cat's Claw (Samento), Olive Leaf

- **Anaplasma**: Colloidal Silver, Noni, Neem

- **Borrelia**: Cat's Claw (Samento), Japanese Knotweed (Resveratrol)

What Is Die-Off?

Before we delve into treatment specifics, I want you to understand the phenomenon of die-off, also known as the Jarisch-Herxheimer or Herxheimer reaction. As these infections die, they release their contents into the body. The immune system sees these as foreign particles and reacts quickly (with cytokines) to remove them from the body. The body then works to remove the infections by sending them through the liver. If the liver's pathways are congested, die-off will be worse.

This reaction is similar to the symptoms you experience when you have the flu. The headaches, fevers, chills, joint pains, fatigue, and body aches you experience when you have the flu are actually from the immune system's *reaction* to the virus, NOT from the virus itself.

When you experience die-off, you may experience symptoms similar to the flu, but some of the time, the symptoms you experience are more infection-specific. For example, *Bartonella* causes symptoms that include fatigue, pain or burning on the bottoms of the feet, sleep problems, anxiety, depression, neck pain, low thyroid, muscle cramps, and headaches. Consequently, die-off usually includes a *worsening* of these symptoms. The intensity can range anywhere from mildly uncomfortable to completely debilitating. The more intense your reaction, the more inflammation you have, and the more stressful this process is on your body and your adrenals.

This process of die-off is the most challenging part of treating these infections. If we didn't have die-off, we could be very aggressive in treating these infections without worry of side effects. Die-off is what usually prevents someone from continuing with a therapy and making progress.

The number-one way to ease the impact of die-off is to *proceed slowly with treatment*. Going slowly allows your detoxification pathways to keep up with the rate of bug death. The image I like to use is that of a bucket being filled with dead bugs and emptied by the liver's detoxification pathways. If the bucket is being filled faster than it is being emptied, it overflows, you get die-off symptoms, and you feel like "crap."

I always want to take my patients through the treatment process as gracefully as possible and with as little die-off as possible. The way to do this is the following:

1. Start low and go slow. Start with the lowest dose and increase slowly.

2. Make sure your hormones are strong and your nutrient replete.

3. Make sure you have good die-off support available. I suggest a process below. If you experience die-off, increase your die-off support until you don't. Use several different kinds of die-off support if you need to.

4. Do not advance your treatment if you have die-off.

5. Stop vitamin D at the first sign of die-off. Vitamin D boosts the immune system's cytokine activity and will make die-off worse.

6. Decrease your treatment dose. If you are unable to mitigate your die-off by increasing die-off support, you will need to decrease your treatment dose. Try to increase your dose again in a week or two.

7. Change the route of administration. If you are taking an oral treatment and you can't find a way to decrease the die-off you are having by decreasing the dose of the treatment and increasing your die-off support, consider using it topically on the bottoms of your feet instead of orally.

8. Do not push through! You may be inclined to think, "No pain, no gain," but that does NOT work in this situation. If you push through, you will drain your hormones (especially cortisol from your adrenal glands), and your healing process will take a lot longer. This process of healing the hormones after destroying them with antibiotics and intense natural treatments is sometimes called "picking up the pieces." I prefer to avoid this painful and costly process. If you follow my advice, you won't have to.

9. Pivot. Stop treating the infection that is causing lots of die-off, and pivot to treat another infection that is easier to treat.

Die-Off Support

At the first sign of die-off, when you feel like you're getting worse after starting an anti-microbial treatment or increasing the dose, follow these instructions:

1. Don't advance to the next dose. DO NOT power through!!

2. Stop taking vitamin D.

3. Start Detox 1, a Byron White Formula that contains the following: Dandelion, Cinnamon, Sarsaparilla, Uva Ursi, Cleavers, Milk Thistle, Barberry, Senna, and Ginger. I recommend 2 drops per night taken with A-BART or whatever antimicrobial you are using. If you have die-off, increase the Detox 1 by 2 drops every day until die-off resolves. Increase Detox 1 by 2 drops every time you increase the anti-microbial to maintain a 2:1 ratio of Detox 1 to the anti-microbial. Some people need a 3:1 or higher ratio to mitigate die off symptoms.

4. If you do not have access to Detox 1, start Sarsaparilla (Smilax): 3 capsules, three times per day and increase by 1 capsule per dose every day until die-off resolves.

5. Start detox baths. Magnesium gel - 2 tsp (or Epsom salt 2 cups), baking Soda 1 cup, hydrogen peroxide - 1/3 cup in hot water. Soak for twenty to thirty minutes every night. Drink plenty of water while bathing. Be careful getting out of the bath because you may feel lightheaded. Consider a lukewarm to cool shower after to rinse off the salts and remove the toxins you eliminated through the skin. Rest for thirty minutes after the bath. (You can also do just Epsom/magnesium salt baths)

If you need more die-off support, proceed with the following:

1. Burbur and Pinella tinctures 30 drops of each in a few ounces of clean water three to four times per day as needed.

2. Parsley tincture 30 drops in a few ounces of clean water three to four times per day as needed.

3. Activated charcoal 6 caps one or two times per day, ninety minutes away from all supplements and food.

4. Sauna for fifteen to thirty minutes two to five times per week as needed.

5. IV Myers (multivitamin) once a week, alternating with IV glutathione once a week. Separated by 48 hours.

6. Alkalization with Optimal Electrolyte 1 scoop once or twice per day

7. Coffee enemas once or twice per day

8. Essiac tea

9. Japanese Knotweed 2000mg up to four times per day

The Wack-A-Mole Effect

Any time you treat an infection, you upset the natural terrain. Our goal is to decrease the burden of the infection and to create a new set point; we are creating a new relationship between the immune system and the infection.

In this process, other infections can emerge and cause symptoms. I call this the Wack-A-Mole Effect. Remember that game of hitting a mole with the rubber mallet and the next one pops up? Yup, that one. This is a very similar effect. During the treatment of one infection, another infection can pop-up.

When this happens, you want to add coverage for the emerging infection as well. Often, the infection that emerges is a yeast or co-infection of *Borrelia*. It is not uncommon to see *Babesia* "pop-out" when treating *Bartonella* or vice versa!

For example, if you're treating *Bartonella* with A-BART (Byron White Formulas), and all of a sudden you start sweating, you're hot all the time, your sleep is getting bad, and you feel anxious and depressed (all symptoms of *Babesia*), you need to treat *Babesia* with A-BAB from Byron White Formulas.

If you cannot tolerate treating both infections concurrently, you must treat the infection that is causing the greatest number of symptoms.

Infections are an enormous drain on the immune system; treating them is essential to recovery from chronic fatigue. Once the immune system uses its resources to combat an infection or two, other opportunistic pathogens can take hold. Even if you have multiple infections, we will conquer them gently and systematically using this protocol.

Reversing Thyroid Disease by Treating *Bartonella*

I love serendipity. One day, my patient Debbie came in for an urgent, same-day appointment. She had just started A-BART to treat her *Bartonella,* and she was having heart palpitations and tremors. I was a bit baffled. These were not typical die-off symptoms from treating *Bartonella*. I asked, "Have you felt this way before?" and she said, "Yes, when I had Graves' disease." Graves' disease causes the body to produce excessive amounts of thyroid hormone. She had been taking thyroid medication for a long time and was doing well. I shrugged my shoulders and said, "Well, let's decrease your thyroid a bit and see if that helps." She did, and it worked like a charm. I was blown away when I began to wean people off of their thyroid medication and reverse their thyroid disease by treating *Bartonella*. I believe *Bartonella* likes to live in the thyroid, and when we start removing it from the body, the thyroid function kicks back in and improves. I find that eighty percent of my patients will wean off of their thyroid medicine completely in three to six months when treated for *Bartonella*.

When patients start to feel hyperthyroid symptoms (tremors, heart palpitations, diarrhea, agitation, anxiety, and insomnia) I recommend they wean off their thyroid medicines. If they are on desiccated thyroid, I recommend they decrease their dose by a half grain every time they have symptoms. If they are on liothyronine, I recommend they decrease by 5 mcg every time they have symptoms. Once they have weaned off desiccated thyroid and liothyronine, I recommend they wean off levothyroxine by 25 mcg every time they have symptoms of too much thyroid.

Summary

Infections are a common cause of fatigue. The declining effectiveness of conventional antibiotics against forever-adapting superbugs is making natural interventions even more of a necessity. In addition to fatigue, patients with chronic infections typically have symptoms of cognitive dysfunction or "brain fog," strange urinary symptoms, cyclical fevers, muscle or joint pain, nerve symptoms (neuropathies), mood issues like depression or anxiety, and autoimmune diseases.

If you suspect an infection, the first step is giving your healthcare provider a good history of your symptoms. Next, is blood testing. The most common stealth infections I see in my fatigue patients are Epstein-Barr virus, *Anaplasma*, *Babesia*, *Bartonella*, *Borrelia* (Lyme), and *Mycoplasma*.

I've had the most success eliminating infections when the *usual suspects* are treated at the same time: heavy metals, chemicals, electromagnetic frequencies, molds, emotions, and food allergies all tax the immune system. The order you go after infections also matters, so I pursue the easiest-to-kill infections and symptomatically significant ones first. Treatments are specific to the type of infection. I also utilize biofilm disruptors, agents that push bacteria out of their cyst form, and treatments to help mitigate die-off.

The Plan

Here are my preferred treatments for infections with specific dosing:

1. Assess for infectious causes of fatigue with symptoms and laboratory testing. Treat based on symptoms more than laboratory results.

2. Start infection-specific treatment with Byron White Formulas. For all of the Byron White Formulas, the dosing ramp-up is going to be the same. You will start with 1 drop per night and increase by 1 drop every seven days up to 30 drops per night. Put the drop in a little water and hold in your mouth for sixty seconds before swallowing. Do not advance if you experience die-off (if you feel worse).

3. Byron White Formulas are typically named for the infection they treat. For *Bartonella*, use A-BART, for *Babesia*, use A-BAB, for Epstein-Barr virus, use A-EB/H6, for *Mycoplasma*, use A-MYCO, and for *Anaplasma*, use A-BIO.

4. Add in one new Byron White Formula with the same ramp-up every three months as long as there is little to no die-off occurring from the other formulas you are taking.

5. After nine months, you can stop treating when the symptoms for a specific infection have been resolved for two months, *and* you have had no die-off for two months. Continue treating until that time.

6. To prevent die-off, start Detox 1 2 drops per night with the above formulas in water. Increase by 1 drop per week up to 31 drops per night. If you experience die-off, increase Detox 1 by 2 drops per night until the die-off resolves. The next time you increase the anti-microbial you are using by 1 drop (i.e. A-BART), increase the Detox 1 as well by 1 drop. Taking more of the Detox 1 helps to clear out any bugs that are dying and opens up the pathways in the liver.

7. To disrupt biofilms: start Interfase Plus 2 capsules two times per day in between meals. NOTE: If you take these supplements with meals, they act as digestive aids and will not disrupt the biofilm.

8. To push *Borrelia* out of its cyst form: start Grapefruit Seed Extract 1 cap two times per day.

There are a lot of nuances to this treatment, so I highly recommend you work with a provider knowledgeable in treating infections and the Byron White Formulas.

If you do not have access to the Byron White Formulas, I recommend the Cowden Support Program. You can find all of the products you will need at Nutramedix.com and the support materials in the member area of our website.

Action Steps

1. Order the new supplements discussed in this chapter. You can find them under the Infection Support and Die-off Support categories in our online store here: us.fullscript.com/welcome/drhirsch.

2. Add your new supplements to your Treatment Schedule.

3. Track your symptoms on the Symptom Calendar

4. Download the Essiac tea brewing instructions and coffee enema protocol from fixyourfatigue.org/members

5. Download the Cowden Support Program summary, schedule and required supplements handouts from the member area.

6. Set alarms on your phone to remind you to take your supplements and when to introduce new treatments.

7. Which infections do you have based on your symptoms? Share with us on the Facebook group at fb.com/groups/fixyourfatigue

8. Ask questions like these in the Facebook group:

   a. *Which infection treatment worked best for you?*

    b. Who in the group has had Bartonella, Babesia, Mycoplasma, etc.?

9. Continue to implement the lifestyle changes you have made and the previous treatments.

10. If you want to hear me talk more about *Bartonella*, tune into the <u>Chronic Lyme Disease Summit #2</u> with Jay Davidson, DC.

11. Congratulations on completing another chapter! Way to go!

12. Get excited to Fix Your Sinus Infections next!

Chapter 18:
Fix Your Sinus Infections

*C*arolyn had chronic sinus congestion and fatigue. Her sinuses had been congested since she was a child. She experienced fullness in her ears, itching in her ear canals, anal itching, skin rashes, constipation, and sugar cravings.

Background

Certain infections thrive in the sinuses, and standard blood tests will not detect them. The most common sinus infections are from mold, yeast, and MARCoNS, or "Multiple Antibiotic Resistant Coagulase Negative Staphylococci." All of these can cause and contribute to fatigue.

MARCoNS is a bacterial sinus infection that can't be treated by the usual antibiotics. It is "resistant" to them. The name MARCoNS is specific to coagulase negative staph. However, it is often used to describe any bacteria that are resistant to multiple antibiotics. We are going to use it in this way.

In a landmark study by the Mayo Clinic in 1999, researchers found that the cause of most chronic sinus infections is an immune system response to fungus. This correlates with my observations as well.

Symptoms

Common symptoms of sinus infections include:

- Fatigue

- Runny nose

- Sinus congestion

- Postnasal drip

- Ear congestion

- Loss of smell

- Sinus headaches

- Facial pain

MARCoNS can produce body-wide symptoms including body aches and debilitating exhaustion. The infection may not necessarily produce traditional sinus symptoms such as a runny nose, sinusitis, or facial pain—in fact, it's been known to grow beyond the sinuses, into the teeth and jaw. MARCoNS are extremely difficult to kill, sometimes colonizing as biofilms. They are also very slow growing, so the standard nasal swab cultures performed by Quest or Lab Corps will not detect these organisms.

Testing

In addition to looking at symptoms, I use a deep nasal swab test to assess for MARCoNS and fungus in the sinus. Symptoms of fungus in the body include skin itching, skin rashes, and sugar cravings. If someone has these symptoms and chronic sinusitis, they most likely have fungi in their sinuses.

Treatment

The treatment for MARCoNS requires a special mix of atypical antibiotics and biofilm disruptors. The antibiotics are Bactroban and Gentamicin, and the biofilm disruptor is EDTA (also a heavy metal chelator). This combination is delivered in the BEG spray. The BEG spray is typically used for one month. If resolution does not occur, I move on to other therapies and come back to the BEG spray. Gentamicin can cause hearing loss, so I don't like to use it for more than a month. Other treatments include colloidal silver nasal spray and sinus ozone. Both of these are broad spectrum anti-microbial agents, so often they will kill infections that the antibiotics will not.

I also use colloidal silver nasal spray for broad-spectrum coverage of any other infections present in the sinuses and Xlear nasal spray to break up biofilm.

The treatment for fungi in the sinuses includes activated charcoal for any mold present, antifungals (natural and pharmaceutical), a biofilm disruptor, and an anti-fungal diet for a minimum of three months.

Summary

The most common infections that we find in the sinuses are mold, yeast, and MARCoNS, or "Multiple Antibiotic Resistant Coagulase Negative Staphylococci." MARCoNS is a bacterial sinus infection that can't be treated by the usual antibiotics.

Common symptoms of sinus infections are a runny nose, nasal congestion, ear congestion, loss of smell, and headaches.

In addition to looking at symptoms, I use a deep nasal swab test to assess for MARCoNS and fungus in the sinus.

The treatment for MARCoNS requires a special mix of atypical antibiotics and biofilm disruptors.

The treatment for fungi in the sinuses includes activated charcoal for any mold present, antifungals (natural and pharmaceutical), a biofilm disruptor, and an anti-fungal diet for a minimum of three months.

The Plan

Clean up your sinuses with this plan based on which infections are present:

For a positive MARCoNS test:

1. Start Sovereign Silver Hydrosol 2 sprays per nostril three times per day

2. Start compounded Bactroban, EDTA, Gentamicin (BEG) spray 1 spray two times per day for one month. Stop immediately if you have any hearing loss. This can be a side effect of the Gentamicin.

3. Start Xlear nasal spray 1-2 sprays in each nostril two to three times per day to break up biofilm.

4. Consider sinus ozone therapy once weekly up to thirty sessions. Ozone is a great anti-microbial.

For mold or yeast in the sinuses:

1. Start Sovereign Silver Hydrosol 2 sprays per nostril three times per day

2. Start Yeast Formula 2 caps three times per day

3. Start Phytostan 2 caps three times per day

4. Start an anti-fungal diet

5. Start activated charcoal 6 capsules before bed ninety minutes after food and supplements.

Action Steps

1. Order the new supplements discussed in this chapter. You can find them under the Sinus Support category in our online store here: us.fullscript.com/welcome/drhirsch

2. Add your new supplements to your Treatment Schedule

3. Track your symptoms on the Symptom Calendar

4. Set alarms on your phone to remind you to take your supplements

5. Download the Antifungal Diet from the member area at fixyourfatigue.org/members.

6. Continue to implement the lifestyle changes you have made and the previous treatments.

7. Congratulations on completing another chapter!

8. Get ready to Fix Your Gut Infections next!

Chapter 19:
Fix Your Gut Infections

Julie had diarrhea for as long as she could remember. She thinks it resulted from exposure to giardia she had one year while she was camping. It had been treated several times, but the diarrhea always came back.

Background

Healing the gut (the gastrointestinal or GI tract) is incredibly important. Your gut is responsible for breaking down your food and absorbing the nutrients. It helps to maintain the health of your immune system and your microbiome (good bugs). Finally, it absorbs water and eliminates waste.

I used to think that if you heal your gut, the rest of your body will follow. I still believe this to an extent, but I have seen quite a few cases where the gut is healed, and the person is not. This is usually due to toxicities from the *usual suspects:* heavy metals, chemicals, molds, infections, allergies, emotions, and electromagnetic frequencies. The converse, however, is true; if you do not heal your gut, you will not heal. You can heal everything else, but if your gut is not healed, you will not resolve your fatigue.

This imbalance in gut bugs (infections) is called dysbiosis. Remember what I told you in the chapter on Stealth Infections: 90 percent of all the cells in our bodies are bacteria, yeast, virus, etc., and only 10 percent are human cells. There is an amazing synergy that exists between these microorganisms and us. We are usually friends until stress or one of the *usual suspects* upsets the balance and causes dysbiosis.

Infections in the gut can be from bacteria, yeast, and parasites and can take place anywhere along the intestinal tract, including the mouth, the stomach, and the small and large intestines.

When the immune system attacks the infection, it causes inflammation, along with pain, and dysfunction, as a byproduct of its normal activity. If the infection is cleared, the inflammation decreases. If the infection is not cleared, the inflammation persists and more pain and dysfunction result. This is chronic inflammation, and we will focus on it in this chapter.

Symptoms

Infections that are found in the gut (along the intestinal track) can cause the following symptoms:

- Fatigue

- Constipation

- Diarrhea

- Reflux

- Bloating

- Flatulence

- Abdominal pain

- Hemorrhoids

- Skin rashes

- Chronic itching (specifically, itching in or around the anus, itching in the ears, and skin itching)

- Sugar cravings (and symptoms worsening with sugar consumption)

- Joint and body pain

- Sinus congestion

- Brain fog

Yeast Infections

Yeast infections (such as candida), mold, or other fungi are very common gut infections. Yeast symptoms are usually fairly distinct: chronic itching (specifically, itching in or around the anus, itching in the ears, and skin itching), sugar cravings (and symptoms worsening with sugar consumption), joint and body pain, skin rashes, sinus congestion, and brain fog. Molds can produce similar symptoms, so if a stool test is negative for yeast, mold is still a possibility.

These yeast symptoms can manifest as vaginal yeast infections, sinus congestion, oral candidiasis (thrush), and intestinal yeast infections.

Small Intestinal Bowel Overgrowth (SIBO)

SIBO is a chronic bacterial infection of the small intestine. The infection is from bacteria that normally live in the large intestine but moved to the small intestine because the environment was conducive to growth. This environment was created from poor food choices, stress, a leaky gut, low stomach acid and digestive enzymes, and other infections.

The main symptoms of SIBO are abdominal bloating (gas), belching, flatulence, abdominal pain, cramps, constipation, diarrhea, heartburn, and nausea.

Consequences of Gut Infections

Infections in the gut will cause inflammation, dysfunction, and eventually increased intestinal permeability or a "leaky gut." The immune system attempts to kill the infection by bringing its immune system components to the fight. As a consequence, it causes swelling, redness, pain, and dysfunction. This is called inflammation. Inflammation of the lining of the intestines because of an infection will damage the connections between the cells and cause them to become permeable or "leaky." This allows foods, toxins, and infections to flow from the intestines into the blood stream. This process triggers the immune system to become more reactive.

A more reactive immune system will result in the following:

- **Food Allergies**: Due to the increase in permeability of the intestines, the immune system detects foreign food particles. It attacks these foods in an attempt to contain and remove them. This causes inflammation, which can produce almost any symptom, including abdominal pain, constipation, diarrhea, headaches, reflux, and others.

- **Autoimmune Diseases:** Infections can trigger the immune system to attack different parts of your body; your joints (as in rheumatoid arthritis), your skin (as in eczema and psoriasis) and your intestines (as in inflammatory bowel disease (IBD)).

- **Skin rashes**: Often when you have an infection in your gut, the immune system will express itself on the skin as a rash.

Other consequences of gut infections include:

- **Nutrient deficiencies**: A decrease in the absorption of nutrients due to leaky gut.

- **Appendicitis**: An infection of the appendix.

- **Diverticulitis:** (an infection in the large intestine).

Testing

Stool tests are invaluable when it comes to sleuthing out gut infections, but they can yield very different results, depending on which laboratory is running the test. Stool testing at your local laboratory will look for the presence of an infection by culture. Functional medicine laboratory stool testing looks for the presence of an infection in stool by culture and PCR (DNA of the infection). Both are dependent on the collection of a good sample that has the infection in it. The functional stool test usually requires collecting the stool for multiple days, which is always a better test. When you collect for multiple days, you have more of a chance of collecting the infection. If the infection lives on the lining of the intestines and doesn't come out in the stool, then it won't be found in a stool test.

I use the GI Effects test by Metametrix (DirectLabs.com), which involves collecting the stool for one or three days. I recommend collecting for three days. This test is a combined culture and DNA (PCR) test that looks for bacterial, fungal, and parasitic gut infections, as well as sensitivities. This means that the lab puts the infection in a petri dish with different herbal and pharmaceutical treatments to determine which herbs and prescriptions will work against which bugs. This is essential for targeting your treatment and avoiding the creation of superbugs through an inappropriate use of antibiotics.

The GI Effects test also tests your microbiome (your probiotic status), your pancreatic enzyme function, your gallbladder function, inflammatory markers, and how well you digest your fats, proteins, and carbohydrates. It's a great test.

SIBO testing can also be done through a breath test (I use Commonwealth Laboratory) to rule out SIBO as a cause of diarrhea, abdominal pain, bloating, and flatulence.

Common Gut Bugs

The most common gut infections (bacteria, yeast, and parasites) I see are:

- **Bacteria**: *Klebsiella, E.coli, Clostridium, Citrobacter, Enterobacter*

- **Yeast**: *Candida Albicans*, Geotrichum, Rhodotorula

- **Parasites**: *Giardia lamblia, Entamoeba histolytica, Blastocystis hominis, Dietamoeba fragilis*

Treatment

Once you figure out that your gut symptoms are coming from an infection and which treatments will work, you can get started.

To treat a bacterial infection, I start with natural antimicrobials (bug killing agents) because of the negative consequences of antibiotics on gut health and our microbiome. Most of us have used antibiotics before (I used them annually when I was a child) and need gut repair. Part of that repair is avoiding further insults from antibiotics.

The herbs that I like to use to treat bacterial infections in the gut include berberine, oregano oil, wormwood (Artemisia), olive leaf, thyme, black walnut bark, barberry root and uva ursi. I have found these herbs in combination in ParaBiotic Plus by Biogenesis, or a combination of GI Microb-X and oregano oil. ParaBiotic Plus dosing is three capsules taken twice daily for three months. GI Microb-X dosing is two capsules taken twice daily. Oregano oil dosing is two capsules two times per day.

Many of these herbs will work against parasites as well, but sometimes prescriptive agents such as metronidazole for Giardia and mebendazole for pinworms, roundworms, or whipworms are necessary.

To treat yeast infections in the gut, you need a four-step approach:

1. **Starve the yeast**: This means an antifungal diet for a minimum of three months. This food plan deprives the yeast of their food – grains, sugars, and carbohydrates. Avoid sugar and artificial sweeteners, white bread, white rice, white pasta, coffee and tea, peanuts, salad dressings, butter, and any food or drink containing yeast. I tell my patients to eat meat and vegetables, no grains, no sugars, and limit fruits. Fruits should only be consumed with proteins.

2. **Push out the yeast**: Probiotics such as *Saccharomyces Boulardii, Bifidobacterium,* and *Lactobacillus* are good for pushing the yeast out of the gut.

3. **Kill the yeast**: On occasion I will use herbal treatments like oregano oil, peppermint, thyme, goldenseal, pau d'arco, caprylic acid, and MCT oil to combat yeast, but I have found that because yeast can be quite stubborn, I frequently need to add in pharmaceuticals such as fluconazole (one capsule daily) and nystatin (two capsules three times daily). Fluconazole is safe to use as long as you take it with Gaia's Daily Liver Formula (two per day) for liver protection and support.

4. **Disrupt the hiding places**: Biofilm disruptors have also proved helpful, such as Interfase Plus (two capsules twice daily, in between meals)

Treatment is generally for three to twelve months or longer depending on how well you can stick to the food plan and how much yeast you have in your body.

To Treat SIBO, I Recommend the Following:

1. **Treat everything else first**: SIBO can be very challenging to treat and often it resolves by treating the *usual suspects.*

2. **A low carbohydrate diet:** I have used the specific carbohydrate diet (SCD), gut and psychology diet (GAPS), FODMAPS diet (a diet that is low in *fermentable oligosaccharides, disaccharides, monosaccharides, and polyols,* which are mainly carbohydrates), and SIBO diet by Dr. Siebecker. I prefer the SIBO diet.

3. **Herbs**: Rifaximin (an antibiotic) will work, but is expensive and has side effects. Several studies have indicated that herbal preparations are as good as antibiotics with fewer side effects. They typically include the following herbs: coptis, Oregon grape, berberine, red thyme oil, oregano oil, sage, and lemon balm. The products that I recommend that contain these herbs are Candibactin-AR and Candibactin-BR.

4. **Probiotics**: *Saccharomyces boulardii* protects beneficial bacteria in the large intestine.

5. **Biofilm disruptors:** to push the SIBO bacteria out of their hiding places.

6. **Hydrochloric acid (HCl):** to enhance stomach acid and create an environment unfriendly to SIBO bacteria.

The Plan

Once you have found the infection in your gut that is contributing to your fatigue, you are ready to treat it.

To treat a bacterial or parasite infection in the gut:

1. Start Parabiotic Plus 3 caps two times per day for three months, then wait a month and recheck your stool test. Make sure you are healing the *usual suspects* as well.

2. Start Interfase Plus 2 caps two times per day in between meals to disrupt the biofilm.

To treat a yeast infection in the gut:

1. Start Yeast Formula 2 caps three times per day

2. Start Phytostan 2 caps three times per day

3. Start anti-fungal diet (also called the anti-candida or anti-yeast diet)

4. Start Saccharomyces Boulardii 1 cap per day

5. Start Interfase Plus 2 caps two times per day in between meals to disrupt the biofilm.

If you're not having success after three months, stop the Yeast Formula and Phytostan and switch to prescription Fluconazole 1 tab/day (take with Gaia Daily Liver Formula 2 per day) and Nystatin 2 caps three times per day.

To treat SIBO:

1. Start the SIBO diet

2. Start Candibactin-AR 2 caps two times per day for one month. If your symptoms persist, continue for two months.

3. Start Candibactin-BR 2 caps two times per day for one month. If your symptoms persist, continue for two months.

4. Start *Saccharomyces boulardii* 1 cap two times per day.

5. Start Interfase Plus 2 caps two times per day in between meals.

6. Start Betaine HCI 1 cap per meal and increase every three days by 1 cap up to 5 caps per meal. When you feel a warmth in your belly or reflux, decrease by 1 cap per meal and continue on that dose until you feel it again. Continue until you wean off the Betaine HCl.

Action Steps

1. Order the new supplements discussed in this chapter. You can find them under the Antimicrobial category in our online store here: us.fullscript.com/welcome/drhirsch

2. Add your new supplements to your Treatment Schedule

3. Track your symptoms on the Symptom Calendar

4. Set alarms on your phone to remind you to take your supplements

5. Download the Antifungal diet packet from the Member area at fixyourfatigue.org/members. This has what to include and exclude from your diet, a shopping list, and meal plans.

6. Download the SIBO diet from the member area.

7. Questions? Ask people in the Facebook group (fb.com/groups/fixyourfatigue) questions like these:

    a. *How many of you were able to get rid of your yeast with the natural versus the prescription antifungals?*

    b. *What's your favorite meal plan on the antifungal diet?*

8. Continue to implement the lifestyle changes you have made and the treatments since then.

9. Way to go! You just completed another chapter! Amazing!

10. Get ready to Fix Your Electromagnetic Frequencies!

Chapter 20:
Fix Your Electromagnetic
Frequencies

*D*onna *was a 60-year-old retired nurse who recently went on a cruise and had a significant exposure to a household cleaner. After this exposure, she started to feel neuropathies (nerve pain) in her feet any time she got near a radio tower or power station. In fact, she could* feel *a power station in her feet before it came into view! The problem got worse, and she began to feel sick in her home. She only felt good in nature.*

Background

We're now living in a sea of electromagnetic frequencies (EMFs). EMFs are generated by anything and everything electrically powered or powered by batteries: computers, cell phones, electric cars, power lines, lights, refrigerator motor, your watch, and all those invisible frequencies like Wi-Fi, Bluetooth, infrared, smart meters, and radio.

Public exposure to electromagnetic radiation has increased dramatically over the past three decades, and now there is an increasing number of studies about a condition known as electromagnetic hypersensitivity syndrome (EHS). EHS is caused by sensitivity to electromagnetic fields, which is a bit like having an electromagnetism "allergy." This is exactly what Donna had.

Our bodies are electrical. We have natural electrical currents moving through our bodies at all times. This electrical activity allows your nervous system to communicate with your brain. The messages conducted via electrical signals from cell to cell in your body control the rhythm of your heartbeat, the movement of blood around your body, and much more.

EMFs can interfere with these currents, disrupting our normal physiology, damaging our DNA (genetic material), and opening the door to pathogens, toxins, and other opportunistic health disruptors. It is hypothesized that the increase in chronic infections we have seen in the last decade is due, in part, to the rise in EMF exposure.

Although many physicians are skeptical about the validity of EHS, the recent science is quite compelling.

- **The BioInitiative Report** with 1,800 published studies can be found at BioInitiative.org. You can download a 1,557-page report of Naval Academy research directed by Dr. Zory R. Glaser, Ph.D. (former advisor to the US FDA).

- **Dr. Magda Havas** (MagdaHavas.com) has collected nearly eight thousand published studies on the negative effects of EMFs on humans and animals.

- **Powerwatch** (powerwatch.org.uk) also has a page on its website devoted to peer-reviewed scientific studies about EMFs.

Science has shown that dirty electricity and other EMFs can interfere with cell physiology, break DNA strands, and disrupt the immune system. The standard electrical frequency used in US homes and offices is 60 hertz. Scientific studies point to a resonance between 60-hertz electricity and the human nervous system, which is disruptive to calcium metabolism. Additional studies have linked EMF exposure with diseases such as Alzheimer's, ADD/ADHD, asthma, cancer, and diabetes.

Symptoms

More research is certainly needed, but I think it's likely these bioelectrical disruptions underlie Electromagnetic Hypersensitivity Syndrome (EHS). The symptoms are highly varied, but in addition to fatigue, the most common symptoms are:

- Fatigue

- Headaches

- Brain fog

- Memory loss

- Sleep disturbances

- Depression and anxiety

- Chronic pain

- Chronic infections

The Top Five Sources of Electromagnetic Radiation and Dirty Electricity

According to EMF expert Vickie Warren, there are five primary sources of EMFs:

1. **Electric fields**: fields emanating from anything with voltage, such as lamps, home electrical wiring, extension cords, electric appliances, automobiles, watches, etc.

2. **Magnetic fields**: These occur where there's an imbalance in the electrical wiring, as well as around electric motors like your refrigerator motor, clock radios, and the smart meter on the outside of your house. Smart meters produce very low-power frequency EMFs, and they communicate by wireless technology.

3. **Power lines**: Above or below ground, these emit high levels of electromagnetic radiation in the radio frequency (RF) range.

4. **Wireless communications**: Cell phones, cell towers, "smart meters" (wireless power meters), wireless routers, cordless phones, and their bases.

5. **Metal plumbing**: Older metal plumbing frequently carries a current.

Let's get Technical (Just for a Second)

This leads us into the subject of dirty electricity or electrosmog. Most modern electric devices now use DC power, so they're equipped with SMPS (switch-mode power supply) converters that convert AC into DC at the outlet, creating high-frequency energy spikes. These spikes produce what's known as dirty electricity.

The problem with dirty electricity is that it does not stay in your wiring—it manifests something called the "skin effect," meaning it travels along the outer skin of the wire and easily passes through walls into our living spaces and our bodies. Ground currents are now practically everywhere carrying dirty electricity into our homes and workplaces.

Among the worse contributors to dirty electricity are compact fluorescent light bulbs (CFLs) because they use "pulsed" energy technology, switching on and off some twenty thousand times per second. This switching activity breaks up the normal 60-hertz sine wave of electrical power into fragments, and then returns these fragments to the electrical system, creating dirty electricity. Dirty electricity can also result from arcing power lines (such as when lines touch trees during storms), and unfiltered cell phone and broadcast frequencies from nearby antennas.

If EMFs are so bad why aren't more people affected?

We are all affected, but not all of us have symptoms. Let me explain. Those with EHS already have a large amount of toxins (heavy metals, chemicals, molds, and infections) in their bodies. Add EMF toxicity onto this large toxin load, and the body becomes overwhelmed, and people become symptomatic. They are the "canaries in the coal mine." Miners used to bring canaries into the mines with them to detect toxic gases. When the canary stopped singing and died, they knew they were being exposed to the gases *even though they didn't feel it or have symptoms.* They knew it was only a matter of time before they would die as well if they didn't leave the mine.

We are all being affected by EMFs, however, depending on our total toxic load and how well we detoxify determines if we have symptoms. As our exposure to toxins increases, we will begin to see more and more people affected by EMFs. It can take between five and twenty years for some people to be affected by this low-level radiation.

My goal in telling you all this bad news is not to make you depressed! Really! It's to make you aware so that you can feel empowered to make changes to your life that can affect your health and the health of your family in a big way. If you're feeling overwhelmed, skip the rest of this chapter and come back to it later when your energy is 7/10, and you have more energy to make some changes.

Testing

You can't test your body directly for EMF toxicity, but you can test your environment and your reaction to EMFs.

First, I highly recommend you test your exposure at home, work and in your car. The best device I've found for this is the Trifield 100XE EMF meter, available from Amazon.

I would also strongly suggest that you simply spend some time in nature and see how you feel. Fatigue is one of many symptoms often lessened by spending time in nature, especially when you are in contact with the earth. If EMFs are triggering your fatigue, then it makes sense that you will feel better spending as much time as possible "off the grid." Your feet have some 1,300 nerve endings per square inch. Spend some time walking barefoot in the grass and see how good you feel. The health benefits are many, and they are significant.

This is also the best way to diagnose yourself with EHS. Since there are no lab tests to run, the diagnosis is made based on your exposure to EMFs. If you feel significantly better away from EMFs, then you may have EHS.

Treatment

Treatment falls into two camps; avoidance and protection. The ideal cure would be moving "off the grid," but obviously not everyone can (or wants to) pick up and move to a remote mountain cabin. If you want to continue to live in modern-day society and use a cell phone and a computer, then you'll need to protect yourself. We can't eliminate all EMF exposure, but there are some practical ways it can be reduced or minimized. The following are a few suggestions to reduce your exposure to dirty electricity in your home and workplace:

1. Minimize the use of devices using SMPS converters

2. Replace dimmer switches with on/off switches

3. Replace compact fluorescent lights with traditional light bulbs

4. Replace smart meters with analog meters

5. Don't allow the installation of smart meters on your property

6. Utilize protective products that help shield you from EMFs in your personal space

7. Remove your phone from your pockets (and bra) as much as possible

8. Turn off Wi-Fi in your home whenever possible (you can use a timer to turn it on and off)

9. Turn off Wi-Fi, mobile data, and Bluetooth on your phone whenever you're not using them

10. Activate the "airplane mode" function on your smartphone if you keep it by your bed at night to reduce your exposure to radiation.

11. If you have EHS, I have found calcium channel blockers, such as hawthorn or magnesium, to be helpful at decreasing symptoms.

There are also some protective devices on the market that I recommend. The products that I have seen work the best come from New Voice for Health (NewVoice.net) and Earth Calm (EarthCalm.com). Both of these companies make necklaces to protect your body and products to protect your space and reduce the EMF exposure from cell phones, laptops, and other electronic devices.

The book *Earthing* by Clinton Ober is about balancing oneself by reconnecting with the earth's electrical potential. Grounding mats, sheets, and blankets are available from Earthing.com. They access the grounding in your house through that little third hole in the electrical outlets.

Unfortunately, governmental agencies, utility companies, and the technology industry continue to downplay the potential harm of electromagnetic fields, turning a blind eye to the burgeoning research. The bottom line is pointedly stated by Martin Blank, PhD (Associate Professor, Department of Physiology and Cellular Biophysics at Columbia University, College of Physicians and Surgeons):

"Cells in the body react to EMFs as potentially harmful, just like to other environmental toxins, including heavy metals and toxic chemicals. The DNA in living cells recognizes electromagnetic fields at very low levels of exposure and produces a biochemical stress response. The scientific evidence tells us that our safety standards are inadequate and that we must protect ourselves from exposure to EMF due to power lines, cell phones and the like, or risk the known consequences. The science is very strong, and we should sit up and pay attention."

Summary

Public exposure to electromagnetic radiation has increased dramatically over the past three decades. Now there is growing awareness about a condition known as electromagnetic hypersensitivity syndrome (EHS), and fatigue is a common symptom. Many physicians are skeptical about the existence of EHS, but the latest research suggests it should not be ignored.

Electromagnetic fields (EMFs) can interfere with the body's natural electrical currents, wreaking havoc with the immune and nervous systems. They can interfere with cell physiology, break DNA strands, and disrupt calcium metabolism. Recent science reveals possible links between EMF exposure and major diseases, including Alzheimer's, ADD/ADHD, asthma, cancer, and diabetes.

Major sources of EMFs include electric household appliances, power meters, power lines, wireless communications, motors, and old metal plumbing. Dirty electricity is especially dangerous because it can penetrate your body via the "skin effect."

The most effective interventions for EHS are spending time in nature, natural calcium channel blockers, and devices that help you reconnect to the earth and protect you from EMFs. EFT can also help reset your electrical currents.

The Plan

EMF toxicity can be a big problem for some people and not for others. However, we are all being exposed, and our health is being negatively affected whether we feel it or not. Please make some of these changes for your health and the health of your family. I have placed these in order of importance:

1. Start removing heavy metals, chemicals, molds, infections, and emotions from your body.

2. Start wearing a necklace (bioTAG) from NewVoice.net, and see how it feels. If you don't feel anything, keep wearing it. If you feel worse wearing it, you probably have EHS. Take it off and spend a few seconds holding it every day (keep it in a separate part of the house if you need to) and slowly build up a tolerance to it. This will help decrease your sensitivity to EMFs. Consider purchasing other products that go on your phone, in your car, on your computers, etc.

3. Start Magnesium Chelate (if you haven't done so already!) 1 cap/night and increase every three nights by 1 capsule until you have soft stools, then back off by 1 capsule. Magnesium is an excellent calcium channel blocker, which may help EHS symptoms.

4. Make sure that when your children are using technology, it is in airplane mode.

5. Remove your phone from your pockets and bra (metal underwire conducts EMFs) whenever possible

6. Turn off your phone at night or activate the airplane mode and keep it far away from your body while you sleep. If you need to keep it on, turn off Wi-Fi, mobile data, and Bluetooth.

7. Start turning off Wi-Fi in your home whenever possible (you can use a timer to turn it on and off). Consider wiring your home for the internet instead of using Wi-Fi.

8. Start turning off Wi-Fi, mobile data, and Bluetooth on your phone whenever you're not using them

9. Start testing your home, and work to see what your exposure is to EMFs using the Trifield 100XE EMF meter.

10. Start spending more time in nature and see how you feel.

11. Start replacing dimmer switches with on/off switches.

12. Start replacing compact fluorescent lights with traditional light bulbs.

13. Start replacing smart meters with analog meters or use a smart meter guard (SmartMeterGuard.com)

14. Start using other protective products that help shield you from EMFs. See EarthCalm.com for their whole house units and NewVoice.net.

15. Start practicing Emotional Freedom Techniques (EFT) to reset your electrical activity. See Stacy's chapter on Fix Your Emotional Health for more information.

Action Steps

1. Order the new products discussed in this chapter to test your home, treat your home, and protect your body and your family.

2. As you implement these reductions in your EMF exposure, track your symptoms on the Symptom Calendar and observe any changes.

3. Questions? Ask people in the Facebook group questions like these:

a. *Has anyone tested a Nissan Leaf's battery for EMF toxicity?*

b. *What is your favorite personal protection product against EMFs? From EarthCalm.com, NewVoice.net or another vendor?*

4. Want more information on EMFs? My friend and colleague Libby Darnell, DC, has done a wonderful job with her four-part EMF blog series here: http://www.revivedliving.com/emf-keeping-your-family-safe-from-electromagnetic-radiation/

5. Learn more about smart meters at StopSmartMeters.org

6. Congratulations on completing the last chapter! You rock!

Stay tuned for what to do next...

Step IV:
Repair

Chapter 21:
Conclusion

Congratulations! You've completed the Fix Your Fatigue Program! You totally did it!

Do you remember when I said that 97 percent of people who purchase programs never finish? You are one of the 3 percent who are taking charge of their lives and saying, "No more fatigue!" You rock!

Let's look at what you've accomplished.

You have started:

- Addressing the foundations (sleep, food, movement, water, and emotional health)

- Replacing your deficiencies in nutrients and hormones

- Removing toxicity from heavy metals, chemicals, molds, infections, EMFs, allergies, and stress

- Repairing your emotions, lymph and detoxification pathways, mitochondria, organs, and your nervous system.

You have also:

- Taken supplements on a daily basis

- Improved your sleep and circadian rhythm

- Changed your diet

- Practiced gratitude (can you feel the difference?)

- Made new friends in the Facebook group

- Improved the quality of your life

- Improved your self-confidence

Way to go!

You may now be asking the following questions:

What now?

At this point, after a minimum of twenty weeks, you are on your way to getting up to full dosing on your therapies. You should be feeling better. Your fatigue is probably not resolved, but your energy should have improved by two to three points. For example, if you came in with an energy level of 2/10, you probably have 4 or 5/10. You're no longer housebound, and you get out into the world for a few hours a day. You can take better care of yourself and your family, and you have hope for a brighter future. Keep on the path, and you will continue to get better!

To stay motivated, please follow me on social media, stay active in our Facebook group, and sign up for our programs. If you start to feel worse, come back to this book or one of our online programs and recommit yourself.

What if I'm not feeling more energetic?

If you're not feeling more energetic, then you may need to do one of the following:

1. **Have patience**: It takes time to remove the heavy metals, chemicals, molds, infections, and emotions from your body. It can take six to twenty-four months for this process to be completed and all of your symptoms to resolve. You'll need to ramp up to full dose on your therapies and make sure you stay consistent on your treatments. This means taking them every day and keeping your supplements filled. Remember, you're looking for more good days and slow-but-steady forward progress. You'll get there!

2. **Treat all causes:** Make sure all of your causes are being treated. Did you notice that you may have treated several causes without an improvement in your symptoms? This is because *all* of the causes need to be treated for the body to reach a state of balance and achieve symptom relief. If you're not having the success you wanted, make sure you addressed all of your causes. You may need to go back and order additional lab testing that you decided to forgo initially. Take a look at *The Plan* and *Action Steps* sections in every chapter. Maybe you need to do that $700 mold test, or maybe you didn't do the stool test. This would be a good time to get those done. Take a look at the Laboratory Testing section in Appendix A for any second and third priorities that may need to get done now.

3. **Change your supplements**: If you chose different supplements for your treatments than the ones that I recommended, they might not have worked. Purchase professional, high-quality supplements and start again.

4. **Set up your day for success**: Take a look at the daily plan you created for yourself at the end of Step I. How close are you to living your ideal schedule? Set a reminder to look at it every month, and make sure you're doing what you need to be doing. Even after you're better, don't forget how you got there. You need to maintain these practices so that you never end up with fatigue again.

5. **Go Paleo**: If you haven't changed your diet yet to a Paleo diet, please go back to the Fix Your Food chapter and do so now. You're going to see amazing things with this diet. It's going to take you to the next level of health. I recommend that you do it with your whole family. The goal is for your diet to be mostly vegetables and meat. Half of your plate at every meal should be vegetables.

6. **Start the food elimination diet**: If you haven't done the food elimination diet yet and your energy is not where you want it to be, go back to the Fix Your Food chapter and start it now. Remove the major food allergens for twenty-one days and then add back in one food every four days and pay attention to your symptoms. Keep track on your Symptom Calendar so you can discern how you are reacting to foods. Remember, you may react to a food immediately after you eat or three days afterward, so pay attention to the possibility of delayed allergies.

7. **Move more**: If your energy is up at 6 or 7/10 and you haven't introduced more exercise and movement in your life, now is the time. Go back to the Fix Your Movement chapter and make a plan. Start low and go slow.

8. **Get more help**: While I've given you all of my tools and protocols, humans are individuals, and there are nuances to every person and every treatment. You may need more help from me or another provider.

How often do I recheck lab work?

I recommend that you recheck your blood work every six months as long as you continue to improve. Recheck every three months if you are not improving or are getting worse.

How long do I continue the supplements?

I recommend that you continue your supplements for at least a year, except for the heavy metal and chemical removal process, which takes two years. After one year, recheck your lab work, and see what you've accomplished. If everything looks good, you can stop one supplement a month. See how you feel and how it affects your lab work. If you feel worse, go back on it. Once you have removed the *usual suspects* (heavy metals, chemicals, molds, infections, allergies, electromagnetic frequencies, and emotions), your body's natural production of hormones should improve, so you should be able to slowly wean off your thyroid, adrenal and sex hormone support. If you're not able to do so, one of the *usual suspects* is still draining your hormones and needs more work.

I want more support; how else can I work with you?

If you'd like more help resolving your fatigue, you can work with me and my team in the following ways:

Take my online courses for more step-by-step support (coming soon!) at FixYourFatigue.org.

Work with me or one of our providers in person or over the phone. You can find my clinic at TheHirschCenter.com.

You may also find practitioners in your area that may be helpful through the following organization's websites. Give them this book!

- IFM.org

- AAEMonline.org

- ACAM.org

- AIHM.org

Hopefully, you feel more energetic and full of hope for the future. You're going to accomplish amazing things in your life. You will look back on your fatigue as just something you had to deal with once upon a time.

I hope this book was helpful for you.

If it was helpful, please add your name to the list of people helped by the Fix Your Fatigue program (goo.gl/forms/ctHqhn1Jnl) and share it with your friends so together we can help 100,000 people resolve their chronic fatigue! We can do it!

Also, if you'd provide me feedback on what was good about the book and what I can do better, I'd really appreciate it!

I'd love to hear about your struggles and successes! Helping people make their lives better is very important to me, so I love to hear about it. I also want to make sure I am providing you the best possible experience on your journey to the health (and the life) of your dreams.

If you have any other questions or comments, please email me at feedback@fixyourfatigue.org.

I feel so blessed to have been part of your journey, and I wish you much success with all of your life goals. Please stay in touch!

If you are a provider and want to know when I'll be offering provider trainings, please email me at the above email address as well.

With heaps of gratitude,

Dr. Evan

P.S. If this book helped you, please let others know that there is a way out of fatigue and post a short review and your success story on Amazon at https://goo.gl/pFFe0y. I will be eternally grateful.

P.P.S. Your support really makes a difference and I read and respond to every review personally so I can make this book even better.

Here are the links if you want to follow me and my work on social media:

Facebook:
https://www.facebook.com/DrEvanHirsch/

Twitter:
https://twitter.com/drevanhirsch

YouTube:
https://www.youtube.com/c/evanhirschmd

LinkedIn:
https://www.linkedin.com/in/drevanhirsch

Google+:
https://plus.google.com/+EvanHirschMD

Appendix A:
Laboratory Testing

In this appendix, I have outlined the following:

- All of the testing (and the lab ranges) that I recommend throughout the book.

- Priorities of what is most important from 1 (highest) to 4 (lowest/not needed).

- Where and how to get it done. If it is not labeled, it may not be available to you through FYF.MyMedLab.com or DirectLabs.com.

- The normal ranges I recommend to help you interpret your labs.

Priority 1:

Blood tests
Labs from FYF.MyMedLab.com or your local medical provider.

Cortisol (not "free cortisol")	15-25 ug/dl
DHEA-S	150-200ug/dl (women), 300-400ug/dl (men)
Vitamin B12	1500-2000 pg/ml
RBC Folate	1500-2000 ng/ml
25 hydroxyvitamin D	60-100 ng/ml
Homocysteine	5-7 umol/L
Magnesium	2.3-2.5 mg/dl
Potassium (K+)	4.0-4.5 mmol/L

Blood Urea Nitrogen (BUN)	6-20 mg/dl
Creatinine (serum)	0.5-0.9 mg/dl
ALT	<34 U/L
AST	<33 U/L
Total bilirubin	<1.2 mg/dl
TIBC	<400 ug/dl
Ferritin	45-55 ng/ml
TSH	0.5-1.5 ulU/ml
Free T4	1.2-2.0 ng/dl
Free T3	3.0-4.0 pg/ml
Anti-thyroglobulin antibody	<115 IU/ml
Anti-thyroid peroxidase antibody	<34 IU/ml
Total testosterone	12-82 ng/dl (women), 500-700 ng/dl (men)
Free testosterone	1.0-2.0ng/dl (women), 8-15 ng/dl (men)
WBC	> 4.0
MCV	90-96 fL

Priority 2:

Blood tests

Labs from FYF.MyMedLab.com or your local medical provider.

Estradiol	<138 pg/ml (postmenopausal)
Estrone	10-55 pg/ml (postmenopausal)
FSH	25-135 pg/ml (postmenopausal)
LH	7-58 mlU/ml (postmenopausal)
Progesterone	< 0.70 ng/ml (postmenopausal)

Sex Hormone Binding Globulin	20-130 nmol/L (women)
Reverse T3	<11 ng/dl
MTHFR A1298C, C677T	negative
Pregnenolone	100-150 ng/dl
Omega-3 index (RBC)	> 9.0 %
Anti-Transglutaminase Ab (tTG IgA, tTG IgG)	Use lab ranges
Anti-Endomysial Ab (Endomysial IGA)	Use lab ranges
Immunoglobulin A (Total IgA)	Use lab ranges
CoQ10	>2.00 ug/ml
Anti-Gliadin Antibodies (Gliadin Ab IgG, IgA)	Use lab ranges

Infection testing in blood: (Medical Diagnostics Laboratory (MDL) or Labcorp) IgG/IgM of the following microorganisms: Epstein-Barr (EBV VCA, EBV EBNA1, EBV-EA-D), Cytomegalovirus, HHV-6, Mycoplasma pneumoniae, Helicobacter pylori, Lyme Disease C6 peptide by ELISA, Lyme Disease by ELISA, Lyme Disease Western Blot, Anaplasma phagocytophilum, Bartonella Henselae, and Babesia microti.

Stool tests

- Infection testing in stool: (Metametrix) GI Effects 3-day stool test (DirectLabs.com).

Priority 3:

Urine tests

- Mold & mycotoxin testing: (RealTime laboratory) Urine mycotoxin testing: (DirectLabs.com).
- Heavy metal testing: (Doctors Data) Urine Toxic Elements (DirectLabs.com).

Priority 4:

Urine tests

- Chemical testing: (Metametrix) Toxic CORE (DirectLabs.com).
- Infection testing in urine: DNA connexions.
- Post-menopausal hormone testing (for patients on BHRT): DUTCH Complete-Precision Analytical Inc. Kit (DirectLabs.com).

Nasal swab

- Sinus (MARCoNS) infection testing: (Microbiology Dx) MARCoNS and fungi sinus testing.

Breath test

- SIBO infection testing: (Commonwealth Laboratories Inc.) breath test.

Blood tests

- Allergy testing: MRT or ALCAT testing (DirectLabs.com).

Saliva tests

- Post-menopausal hormone testing (for patients not on BHRT): (ZRT) Hormone Saliva Test (FYF.MyMedLab.com).

References

Chapter 1: Causes of Fatigue

1. https://www.cdc.gov/cfs/diagnosis/index.html
2. https://www.cdc.gov/cfs/general/index.html)
3. Teitelbaum J., Bird B. Effective treatment of severe chronic fatigue: a report of a series of 64 patients. J Musculoskelet Pain.. 1995;3: 91-110.
4. Teitelbaum J.E., Bird B., Greenfield R.M., et al: Effective treatment of CFS and FMS: a randomized, double-blind placebo controlled study. J Chronic Fatigue Syndr. 2001;8. www.Vitality101. com) 3– 24.
5. Demitrack M.A., Dale K., Straus S.E., et al. Evidence for impaired activation of the hypothalamic-pituitary-adrenal axis in patients with chronic fatigue syndrome. J Clin Endocrinol Metab.. 1991;73: 1223-1234.
6. Teitelbaum J. Estrogen and testosterone in CFIDS/ FMS. From Fatigued to Fantastic Newsletter. 1997. Feb: 1– 8
7. Behan P.O. Postviral fatigue syndrome research. In: Hyde B., Goldstein J., Levine P., editors. The Clinical and Scientific Basis of Myalgic Encephalitis and Chronic Fatigue Syndrome. Ottawa: Nightingale Research Foundation; 1992: 238.
8. Teitelbaum J. Mitochondrial dysfunction. From Fatigued to Fantastic Newsletter. 1997;1: 1-8.
9. Humulus lupus [monograph]. Altern Med Rev. 2003;8: 190-192. 17 Cronin J.R. Passionflower: reigniting male libido and other potential uses. Altern Complement Ther. 2003: 89-92.
10. Faglia G., Bitensky L., Pinchera A., et al. Thyrotropin secretion in patients with central hypothyroidism: evidence for reduced biological activity of immunoreactive thyrotropin. J Clin Endocrinol Metab. 1979;48: 989-998.

11. Skinner G.R., Holmes D., Ahmad A., et al. Clinical response to thyroxine sodium in clinically hypothyroid but biochemically euthyroid patients. J Nutr Environ Med. 2000;10: 115-125.

12. Asvold B., Bjøro T., Nilsen T.I., et al. Thyrotropin levels and risk of fatal coronary heart disease: the HUNT study. Arch Intern Med. 2008;168: 855-860.

13. Nordyke R.A., Reppun T.S., Madanay L.D., et al. Alternative sequences of thyrotropin and free thyroxine assays for routine thyroid function testing. Quality and cost. Arch Intern Med. 1998;158: 266-272.

14. Griep E.N., Boersma J.N., de Kloet E.R. Altered reactivity of the hypothalamic-pituitary axis in the primary fibromyalgia syndrome. J Rheumatol. 1993;20: 469-474.

15. McKenzie R., O'Fallon A., Dale J., et al. Low-dose hydrocortisone for treatment of chronic fatigue syndrome: a randomized controlled trial. JAMA. 1998;280: 1061-1066.

16. Teitelbaum J.E., Bird B., Weiss A., et al. Low dose hydrocortisone for chronic fatigue syndrome. JAMA. 1999;281: 1887-1888.

17. Holtorf K. Diagnosis and treatment of hypothalamic-pituitary-adrenal (HPA) axis dysfunction in patients with chronic fatigue syndrome (CFS) and fibromyalgia (FM). J Chronic Fatigue Syndr. 2008;14: 1-14.

18. Rakel, David. Integrative Medicine E-Book (Rakel, Integrative Medicine) (Kindle Locations 39119-39121). Elsevier Health Sciences. Kindle Edition.

Chapter 3: Fix Your Sleep

19. Ding D et al. "Traditional and Emerging Lifestyle Risk Behaviors and All-Cause Mortality in Middle-Aged and Older Adults: Evidence from a Large Population-Based Australian Cohort" Plos Medicine December 2015 http://dx.doi.org/10.1371/journal.pmed.1001917

20. Xie L et al. "Sleep Drives Metabolite Clearance from the Adult Brain." Science October 18, 2013; 342(6156):373-377 DOI: 10.1126/science.1241224

21. Healthy Sleep: Sleep and Disease Risk, Harvard

22. NIGMS: Circadian Rhythms Fact Sheet. http://www.nigms.nih.gov/Education/Pages/Factsheet_CircadianRhythms.aspx

23. Youngken H. Textbook of Pharmacognosy, 6th ed. Philadelphia: Blakiston; 1948.

24. Schultz V., Hansel R., Tyler V.E. Restlessness and sleep disturbances. In Rational Therapy: A Physicians' Guide to Herbal Medicine. Berlin: Springer-Verlag; 1998.

25. Reichert R. Valerian. Q Rev Nat Med. 1998: 207-215. Fall

26. 19. R. Cluydt, "Insomnia Treatment: A Postgraduate Medicine Special Report," 114–123.

27. D. Buchwald, R. Pascualy, and C. Bombardier, et al., "Sleep Disorders in Patients with Chronic Fatigue," Clin Infect Dis 1994; 18 (supplement 1): S68–S72.

28. R. P. Millman, "Do You Ever Take a Sleep History?" Annals of Internal Medicine 131 (7) (October 1999): 535–536.

29. E. G. Lutz, "Restless Legs, Anxiety and Caffeinism," Journal of Clinical Psychiatry 39 (9) (September 1978): 693–698.

30. Teitelbaum, Jacob. From Fatigued to Fantastic: A Clinically Proven Program to Regain Vibrant Health and Overcome Chronic Fatigue and Fibromyalgia New, revised third edition. Penguin Group.

Chapter 4: Fix Your Water

31. Chronic Fatigue In-Depth Report. http://www.nytimes.com/health/guides/disease/chronic-fatigue-syndrome/print.html

32. 75% of Americans May Suffer From Chronic Dehydration, According to Doctors.

http://www.medicaldaily.com/75-americans-may-suffer-chronic-dehydration-according-doctors-247393

33. D'Anci K.E., Vibhakar A., Kanter J.H., et al. Voluntary dehydration and cognitive performance in trained college athletes. Percept Mot Skills. 2009;109: 251-269.

34. Edmonds C.J., Jeffes B. Does having a drink help you think? 6– 7-year-old children show improvements in cognitive performance from baseline to test after having a drink of water. Appetite. 2009;53: 469-472.

35. Chung B., Parekh U., Sellin J. Effect of increased fluid intake on stool output in normal healthy volunteers. J Clin Gastroenterol.. 1999;28: 29-32.

36. Anti M., Pignataro G., Armuzzi A., et al. Water supplementation enhances the effect of high-fiber diet on stool frequency and laxative consumption in adult patients with functional constipation. Hepatogastroenterology.. 1998;45: 727-732.

37. Rakel, David. Integrative Medicine E-Book (Rakel, Integrative Medicine) (Kindle Locations 37783-37787). Elsevier Health Sciences. Kindle Edition.

Chapter 5: Fix Your Food

38. Ji, S. "The Dark Side of Wheat—New Perspectives on Celiac Disease and Wheat Intolerance,"

39. Gunnars, K. (January 2013) "How Sugar Hijacks Your Brain And Makes You Addicted." http://authoritynutrition.com/how-sugar-makes-you-addicted/

40. Joneja J.V. Dietary Management of Food Allergy and Intolerance, 2nd ed. Vancouver, BC: Hall Publishing Group; 1998.

41. Arora D., Kumar M. Food allergies: leads from Ayurveda. Indian J Med Sci.. 2003;57: 57-63.

42. Kristjánsson G, Högman M, Venge P, et al Gut mucosal granulocyte activation precedes nitric oxide production:

studies in coeliac patients challenged with gluten and corn Gut 2005;54:769-774.

43. Zopf Y., Baenkler H.W., Silbermann A. The differential diagnosis of food intolerance. Dtsch Arztebl.. 2009;106: 359-370.

44. Degaetani M.A., Crowe S.E. A 41-year-old woman with abdominal complaints: is it food allergy or food intolerance? How to tell the difference. Clin Gastroenterol Hepatol.. 2010;8: 755-759.

45. Sampson H.A. Update on food allergy. J Allergy Clin Immunol.. 2004;113: 805-819.

46. Sampson H.A., Sicherer S.H., Birnbaum A.H. AGA technical review on the evaluation of food allergy in gastrointestinal disorders. Gastroenterology.. 2001;120: 1026-1040.

47. Bjarnason I., MacPherson A., Hollander D. Intestinal permeability: an overview. Gastroenterology.. 1995;108: 1566-1581.

48. Wald A., Rakel D. Behavioral and complementary approaches for the treatment of irritable bowel syndrome. Nutr Clin Pract.. 2008;23: 284-292.

49. Hollander D. Intestinal permeability, leaky gut, and intestinal disorders. Curr Gastroenterol Rep.. 1999;1: 410-416.

50. Nejdfors P., Ekelund M., Westrom B.R. Intestinal permeability in humans is increased after radiation therapy. Dis Colon Rectum.. 2000;43: 1582-1587.

51. Iwata H., Matsushi M., Nishikimi N. Intestinal permeability is increased in patients with intermittent claudication. J Vasc Surg.. 2000;31: 1003-1007.

52. Yacyshyn B., Meddings J., Sadowski D. Multiple sclerosis patients have peripheral blood CD45RO + B cells and increased intestinal permeability. Dig Dis Sci.. 1996;41: 2493-2498.

53. Keshavarzian A., Holmes E.W., Patel M. Leaky gut in alcoholic cirrhosis: a possible mechanism for alcohol-

induced liver damage. Am J Gastroenterol.. 1999;94: 200-207.

54. Reichelt K.L., Knivsberg A.M. The possibility and probability of a gut-to-brain connection in autism. Ann Clin Psychiatry.. 2009;21: 205-211.

55. Genuis S.J. Sensitivity-related illness: the escalating pandemic of allergy, food intolerance, and chemical sensitivity. Sci Total Environ.. 2010;408: 6047-6061.

56. Rakel, David. Integrative Medicine E-Book (Rakel, Integrative Medicine) (Kindle Locations 65090-65097). Elsevier Health Sciences. Kindle Edition.

Chapter 6: Fix Your Movement

57. U.S. Department of Health and Human Services. Physical Activity and Health: A Report of the Surgeon General. Atlanta: Centers for Disease Control and Prevention; 1996.

58. U.S. Preventive Services Task Force. Guide to Clinical Preventive Services, 2nd ed., Baltimore: Williams & Wilkins, 1996.

59. Kligman E.W., Hewitt M.J., Crowell D.L. Recommending exercise to healthy older adults: the preparticipation evaluation and exercise prescription. Physician Sportsmed.. 1999;27: 42-62.

60. American College of Sports Medicine Position Stand. Exercise and physical activity for older adults. Med Sci Sports Exerc. 2009;41: 1510-1530.

61. American College of Sports Medicine Position Stand. Appropriate physical activity intervention strategies for weight loss and prevention of weight regain for adults. Med Sci Sports Exerc. 2009;41: 459-471.

62. Lohman T.G. Advances in Body Composition Assessment. Champaign, IL: Human Kinetics; 1992.

63. Lohman T.G., Roche A.F., Martorell R. Anthropometric Standardization Reference Manual. Champaign, IL: Human Kinetics; 1988.

64. Lohman T.G., Houtkooper L., Going S.B. Body fat measurement goes high-tech: not all are created equal. ACSM Health Fitness J.. 1997;1: 30-35.

65. American College of Sports Medicine. Position Stand. Quantity and quality of exercise for developing and maintaining cardiorespiratory, musculoskeletal, and neuromotor fitness in apparently healthy adults: guidance for prescribing exercise. Med Sci Sports Exerc.. 2011;43: 1334-1359.

66. Borg G.A. Psychophysical bases of perceived exertion. Med Sci Sports Exerc.. 1982;14: 377-381.

67. Robertson R.J., Goss F.L., Andreacci J.L. Validation of the children's OMNI RPE scale for stepping exercise. Med Sci Sports Exerc.. 2005;37: 290-298.

68. Rakel, David. Integrative Medicine E-Book (Rakel, Integrative Medicine) (Kindle Locations 66708-66714). Elsevier Health Sciences. Kindle Edition.

Chapter 7: Fix Your Emotional Health

69. Nixon PG. The human function curve - a paradigm for our times. Act Nerv Super (Praha). 1982;Suppl 3(Pt 1):130-3.

70. Hockenbury & Hockenbury (2007). Discovering Psychology: Fourth Edition. New York: Worth Publishers, Inc.

71. Myers, D. G. (2004). Theories of Emotion. Psychology: Seventh Edition, New York, NY: Worth Publishers.

72. G. L. Macklem, Practitioner's Guide to Emotion Regulation in School-Aged 13 Children. Ó Springer 2008

73. "Relationship of Childhood Abuse and Household Dysfunction to Many of the Leading Causes of Death in Adults," published in the American Journal of Preventive Medicine in 1998, Volume 14, pages 245–258.

74. Heim C, Wagner D, Maloney E, Papanicolaou DA, Solomon L, Jones JF, Unger ER, Reeves WC. Early Adverse Experience and Risk for Chronic Fatigue

SyndromeResults From a Population-Based Study. *Arch Gen Psychiatry.* 2006;63(11):1258-1266. doi:10.1001/archpsyc.63.11.1258

75. National Scientific Council on the Developing Child. (2005/2014). Excessive Stress Disrupts the Architecture of the Developing Brain: Working Paper 3. Updated Edition. http://www.developingchild.harvard.edu

76. Masten AS. "Ordinary Magic: Resilience Processes in Development," American Psychologist (March 2001): Vol. 56, No. 3, pp. 227-38.

77. National Scientific Council on the Developing Child. (2015). Supportive Relationships and Active Skill-Building Strengthen the Foundations of Resilience: Working Paper 13. http://www.developingchild.harvard.edu

78. Sansone RA, Sansone LA. Gratitude and Well Being: The Benefits of Appreciation. Psychiatry (Edgmont). 2010;7(11):18-22.

79. Emmons, R. A., & McCullough, M. E. (2004). The psychology of gratitude. Oxford University Press.

80. Emmons, R. A. (2007). Thanks!: How the new science of gratitude can make you happier. Houghton Mifflin Harcourt.--

81. Neff, K. D. (2011). Self-compassion, self-esteem, and well-being. Social and personality psychology compass, 5(1), 1-12.

82. Neff, K. D. (2011). Self-compassion, self-esteem, and well-being. Social and personality psychology compass, 5(1), 1-12.

83. Pennebaker, J. W., Zech, E., & Rimé, B. (2001). Disclosing and sharing emotion: Psychological, social, and health consequences. Handbook of bereavement research: Consequences, coping, and care, 517-543.

84. Lutz, A., Brefczynski-Lewis, J., Johnstone, T., & Davidson, R. J. (2008). Regulation of the neural circuitry of emotion by compassion meditation: effects of meditative expertise. PloS one, 3(3), e1897.

85. Lutz, A., Brefczynski-Lewis, J., Johnstone, T., & Davidson, R. J. (2008). Regulation of the neural circuitry of emotion by compassion meditation: effects of meditative expertise. PloS one, 3(3), e1897.

86. Tang, Y. Y., Ma, Y., Wang, J., Fan, Y., Feng, S., Lu, Q., ... & Posner, M. I. (2007). Short-term meditation training improves attention and self-regulation. Proceedings of the National Academy of Sciences, 104(43), 17152-17156.

87. Hill, C. L., & Updegraff, J. A. (2012). Mindfulness and its relationship to emotional regulation. Emotion, 12(1), 81.

88. Church, D., Yount, G., & Brooks, A. J. (2012). The effect of emotional freedom techniques on stress biochemistry: a randomized controlled trial. The Journal of nervous and mental disease, 200(10), 891-896.

89. Church, D., Hawk, C., Brooks, A. J., Toukolehto, O., Wren, M., Dinter, I., & Stein, P. (2013). Psychological trauma symptom improvement in veterans using emotional freedom techniques: a randomized controlled trial. The Journal of nervous and mental disease, 201(2), 153-160.

90. Childre, D., & McCraty, R. (2002). Appreciative Heart: The Psychophysiology of Positive Emotions and Optimal Functioning, The.

91. Heller, L., & LaPierre, A. (2012). Healing developmental trauma: How early trauma affects self-regulation, self-image, and the capacity for relationship. North Atlantic Books.

92. Coubard, O. A. (2015). Eye movement desensitization and reprocessing (EMDR) re-examined as cognitive and emotional neuroentrainment. Frontiers in human neuroscience, 8, 1035.

93. Barstow, C. (1985). An overview of the Hakomi method of psychotherapy. In Hakomi Forum. Hakomi Institute.

94. Johnston, S. J., Boehm, S. G., Healy, D., Goebel, R., & Linden, D. E. (2010). Neurofeedback: A promising tool for the self-regulation of emotion networks. Neuroimage, 49(1), 1066-1072.

95. Yucha, C., & Montgomery, D. (2008). Evidence-based practice in biofeedback and neurofeedback. Wheat Ridge, CO: AAPB.

96. Fisher, S. F. (2014). Neurofeedback in the treatment of developmental trauma: Calming the fear-driven brain. WW Norton & Company.

97. Halberstein, R., DeSantis, L., Sirkin, A., Padron-Fajardo, V., & Ojeda-Vaz, M. (2007). Healing with Bach® flower essences: testing a complementary therapy. Complementary health practice review, 12(1), 3-14.

98. McCann, T. (2011). An evaluation of the effects of a training programme in Trauma Release Exercises on Quality of Life (Doctoral dissertation, University of Cape Town).

Chapter 8: Fix Your Adrenals

99. Wilson, James L. Adrenal Fatigue: The 21st Century Stress Syndrome. Petaluma, CA: Smart Publications, 2001.

100. Stop the Thyroid Madness (STTM): Seven Stages of Adrenal Issues

101. Jefferies, William M. Safe Uses of Cortisol. Charles C Thomas Pub Ltd, 2004. Print.

102. Stein-Behrins B.A., Sapolsky R. Stress, glucocorticoids and aging. Aging Clin Exp Res. 1992;4: 197-210.

103. Sapolsky R. Stress, the Aging Brain, and the Mechanisms of Neuron Death. Cambridge, MA: Bradford; 1992. 14 McEwen B.S., Sapolsky R.M. Stress and cognitive function. Curr Opin Neurobiol. 1995;5: 205-216. 15 Sapolsky R. Glucocorticoids, hippocampal damage and the glutamatergic synapse. Proc Brain Res. 1992;86: 13-23. 16 Crowe M., Andel R., Pedersen N.L., Gatz M. Do work-related stress and reactivity to stress predict dementia more than 30 years later? Alzheimer Dis Assoc Disord. 2007;21: 205-209.

104.   Newcomer J.W., Selke G., Melson A.K., et al. Decreased memory performance in healthy humans induced by stress-level cortisol treatment. Arch Gen Psychiatry. 1999;56: 527-533.

105.   Wilson R.S., Evans D.A., Bienias J.L., et al. Proneness to psychological distress is associated with risk of Alzheimer's disease. Neurology. 2003;61: 1479-1485.

106.   Peavy G.M., Lange K.L., Salmon D.P., et al. The effects of prolonged stress and APOE genotype on memory and cortisol in older adults. Biol Psychiatry. 2007;62: 472-478.

Chapter 9: Fix Your Thyroid

107.   American Thyroid Association General Information/Fact Sheet

108.   Kohrle, J. Selenium and the Thyroid. Curr. Opin Endocrinol Diabetes Obes. 2015 Oct.;22(5):392-401 doi: 10.1097/MED.0000000000000190.

109.   Brent, G. A. Environmental Exposures and Autoimmune Thyroid Disease. Thyroid. 2010 July;20(7):755-761 doi: 10.1089/thy.2010.1636 PMCID: PMC2935336

110.   Biology of Belief. Bruce Lipton, PhD

111.   Iodine: Why You Need It, Why You Can't Live Without It. David Brownstein, MD.

112.   Rose S.R. Improved diagnosis of mild hypothyroidism using time-of-day normal ranges for thyrotropin. J Pediatr. 2010;157: 662-667.

113.   Surks M.I., Ortiz E., Daniels G.H., et al. Subclinical thyroid disease: scientific review and guidelines for diagnosis and management. JAMA. 2004;291: 228-238.

114.   Roberts C.G.P., Ladenson P.W. Hypothyroidism. Lancet. 2004;363: 793-803.

115.   Biondi B., Cooper D.C. The clinical significance of subclinical thyroid dysfunction. Endocr Rev. 2008;29: 76-131.

116.   Smallridge R.C. Thyroid function tests. In: Becker K.L., Bilezikian J.P., Bremner W.J., et al, editors. Principles and Practice of Endocrinology and Metabolism. 3rd ed. Philadelphia: Lippincott Williams & Wilkins; 2001: 330.

117.   Shapiro L.E., Surks M.I. Hypothyroidism. In: Becker K.L., Bilezikian J.P., Bremner W.J., et al, editors. Principles and Practice of Endocrinology and Metabolism. 3rd ed. Philadelphia: Lippincott Williams & Wilkins; 2001: 450.

118.   Villar H.C., Saconato H., Valente O., et al. Thyroid hormone replacement for subclinical hypothyroidism. Cochrane Database Syst Rev. (3): 2007. CD003419

119.   Rodondi N., den Elzen W., Bauer D., et al. Subclinical hypothyroidism and the risk of coronary heart disease and mortality. JAMA. 2010;304: 1365-1374.

Chapter 10: Fix Your Sex Hormones

120.   US Department of Health and Human Services, Office on Women's Health: PMS Fact Sheet

121.   US Department of Health and Human Services, Office on Women's Health: PCOS Fact Sheet

122.   Tartavoulle, T.M. Low T Prevalence. Journal for Nurse Practitioners 2012;8(10):778-786

123.   Shores, M.M. et al. Testosterone treatment and mortality in men with low testosterone levels. J Clin Endocrinol Metab. 2012 Jun;97(6):2050-8 doi: 10.1210/jc.2011-2591

124.   State of the Science of Endocrine Disrupting Chemicals – 2012. World Health Organization and UNEP

125.   Environmental Working Group: Dirty Dozen Endocrine Disruptors

126.   C. Guilleminault, L. Palombini, D. Poyares, et al., "Chronic Insomnia, Postmenopausal Women, and SDB, Part 2: Comparison of Nondrug Treatment Trials in

Normal Breathing and UARS Postmenopausal Women Complaining of Insomnia," J Psychosom Res 2002; 53: 617–623.

127.   Teitelbaum, Jacob. From Fatigued to Fantastic: A Clinically Proven Program to Regain Vibrant Health and Overcome Chronic Fatigue and Fibromyalgia New, revised third edition. Penguin Group.

Chapter 11: Fix Your Nutrients

128.   Dr. Michael F. Holick Official website
129.   Mercola, J. (February 2015) "Great Reasons to Eat More Sprouts" Mercola.com
130.   Kresser C. (March 2012) "The Little Known (but Crucial) Difference Between Folate and Folic Acid" Chriskresser.com
131.   R. M. Marston and B. B. Peterkin, "Nutrient Content of the National Food Supply," National Food Review, Winter 1980, pp. 21–25.
132.   R. M. Marston and B. B. Peterkin, op. cit.; and J. H. Nelson, "Wheat: Its Processing and Utilization," American Journal of Clinical Nutrition 41, supplement (May 1985): 1070–1076.
133.   H. A. Schroeder, "Losses of Vitamins and Trace Minerals Resulting from Processing and Preservation of Foods," American Journal of Clinical Nutrition 24 (5) (May 1971): 562–573.
134.   H. C. Trowell, ed., Western Diseases: Their Emergence and Prevention (Cambridge, MA: Harvard University Press, 1981).
135.   S. B. Eaton and N. Konner, "Paleolithic Nutrition. A Consideration of Its Nature and Current Implications," New England Journal of Medicine 312 (5) (31 January 1985): 283–289.
136.   W. Mertz, ed., "Beltsville 1 Year Dietary Intake Survey," American Journal of Clinical Nutrition 40, supplement (December 1984): 1323–1403.

137. B. Bartali et al., "Low Micronutrient Levels as a Predictor of Incident Disability in Older Women," Arch Intern Med 2006; 166: 2335–2340.

138. "The Relationship Between Dietary Intake and the Number of Teeth in Elderly Japanese Subjects," Gerodontology 2005; 22 (4): 211–218.

139. S. Ozgocmen, H. Ozyurt, S. Sogut, O. Akyol, O. Ardicoglu, and H. Yildizhan, "Antioxidant Status, Lipid Peroxidation and Nitric Oxide in Fibromyalgia: Etiologic and Therapeutic Concerns," Rheumatol Int 2005 November 10; 1–6 (E-pub ahead of print).

140. S. Hercberg et al., Arch Intern Med 2004; 164: 2335–2342.

141. R. van Leeuwen, S. Boekhoorn, et al., "Dietary Intake of Antioxidants and Risk of Age-Related Macular Degeneration," JAMA 2005; 294 (24): 3101–3107.

142. http://www.medscape.com/viewarticle/520823 20. I. S. Kwun, K. H. Park, et al., "Lower Antioxidant Vitamins (A, C and E) and Trace Minerals (Zn, Cu, Mn, Fe and Se) Status in Patients with Cerebrovascular Disease," Nutr Neurosci, 2005; 8 (4): 251–257. 21. J. A. Pasco, M. J. Henry, et al., "Antioxidant Vitamin Supplements and Markers of Bone Turnover in a Community Sample of Nonsmoking Women," J Womens Health (Larchmont), 2006; 15 (3): 295–300.

143. S. Das, R. Ray, et al., "Effect of Ascorbic Acid on Prevention of Hypercholesterolemia Induced Atherosclerosis," Mol Cell Biochem 2006 February 14.

144. http://www.medicalnewstoday.com/medicalnews.php?newsid=40914

145. S. Sasazuki, S. Sasaki, et al., "Effects of Vitamin C on Common Cold: Randomized Controlled Trial," European Journal of Clinical Nutrition, August 24, 2005 (e-published ahead of print).

146. Y. Miyake, S. Sasaki, et al., "Dietary Folate and Vitamins B12, B6, and B2 Intake and the Risk of Postpartum Depression in Japan: The Osaka Maternal

and Child Health Study," J Affect Disord 2006 June 29 (E-published ahead of print).

147. http://www.my.webmd.com/content/Article/90/10 0791.htm

148. Y. Osono, N. Hirose, K. Nakajima, and Y. Hata, "The Effects of Pantethine on Fatty Liver and Fat Distribution," J Atheroscler Thromb 2000; 7 (1): 55–58.

149. C. H. Cheng, S. J. Chang, et al., "Vitamin B6 Supplementation Increases Immune Responses in Critically Ill Patients," Eur J Clin Nutr 2006; 60 (10): 1207–1213.

150. P. T. Lin, C. H. Cheng, et al., "Low Pyridoxal 5´Phosphate Is Associated with Increased Risk of Coronary Artery Disease," Nutrition 2006 October 9 (E-published ahead of print).

151. http://www.medscape.com/viewarticle/506337; Gastroenterology June 2005; 128: 1830–1837.

152. J. Lindenbaum, E. B. Healton, D. G. Savage, et al., "Neuropsychiatric Disorders Caused by Cobalamin Deficiency in the Absence of Anemia or Macrocytoses," New England Journal of Medicine 318 (26) (30 June 1988): 1720–1728.

153. J. Lindenbaum, I. H. Rosenberg, P. W. Wilson, et al., "Prevalence of Cobalamin Deficiency in the Framingham Elderly Population," American Journal of Clinical Nutrition 60 (1) (July 1994): 2–11.

154. W. S. Beck, "Cobalamin and the Nervous System," editorial, New England Journal of Medicine 318 (1988): 1752–1754.

155. D. S. Karnaze and R. Carmel, "Low Serum Cobalamin Levels in Primary Degenerative Dementia: Do Some Patients Harbor Atypical Cobalamin Deficiency States?" Archives of Internal Medicine 147 (3) (March 1987): 429–431.

156. B. Regland, M. Andersson, L. Abrahamsson, et al., "Increased Concentrations of Homocysteine in the Cerebrospinal Fluid in Patients with Fibromyalgia and

Chronic Fatigue Syndrome," Scandinavian Journal of Rheumatology 26 (4) (1997): 301–307.

157.   V. Lerner, "Vitamin B12 and Folate Serum Levels in Newly Admitted Psychiatric Patients," Clin Nutr, 2006 February; 25 (1): 60–67.

158.   E-published 2005 October 10. 44868 (6/2006).

159.   R. A. Dhonukshe-Rutten et al. "Homocysteine and Vitamin B12 Status Relate to Bone Turnover Markers, Broadband Ultrasound Attenuation, and Fractures in Healthy Elderly People," J Bone Miner Res 2005 June; 20 (6): 921–929; and M. S. Morris, P. F. Jacques, and J. Selhub, "Relation Between Homocysteine and B-vitamin Status Indicators and Bone Mineral Density in Older Americans," Bone 2005; 37 (2).

160.   J. Robertson, F. Iemolo, et al., "Vitamin B12, Homocysteine and Carotid Plaque in the Era of Folic Acid Fortification of Enriched Cereal Grain Products," CMAJ 2005; 172 (12): 1569–1573.

161.   D. E. Diaz, A. M. Tuesta, M. D. Ribo, et al., "Low Levels of Vitamin B12 and Venous Thromboembolic Disease in Elderly Men," Journal of Internal Medicine 2005; 258 (3): 244–249.

162.   M. Lajous et al., "Folate, Vitamin B6, and Vitamin B12 Intake and the Risk of Breast Cancer Among Mexican Women," Cancer Epidemiology Biomarkers & Prevention, Vol. 15, March 2006, 443–448.

163.   http://www.latimes.com/news/nationworld/nation/wire/ats-ap_health10jun 20,1,7209352.story?coll=sns-ap-tophealth&ctrack=1&cset=true

164.   G. Ravaglia, P. Forti, et al., "Homocysteine and Folate as Risk Factors for Dementia and Alzheimer's Disease," American Journal of Clinical Nutrition 2005; 82 (3): 636–643; and http://www.lef.org/protocols/prtcl-006.shtml

165.   S. Kono and K. Chen, "Genetic Polymorphisms of Methylenetetrahydrofolate Reductase and Colorectal

Cancer and Adenoma," Cancer Science 2005; 96 (9): 535–542.

166. M. F. Holick, "High Prevalence of Vitamin D Inadequacy and Implications for Health," Mayo Clin Proc 2006; 81 (3): 353–373.

167. http://www.medscape.com/viewarticle/529426; and E. Giovannucci, Y. Liu, E. B. Rimm, B. W. Hollis, C. S. Fuchs, M. J. Stampfer, and W. C. Willett, "Prospective Study of Predictors of Vitamin D Status and Cancer Incidence and Mortality in Men," J Natl Cancer Inst 2006; 98: 451–459.

168. M. Berwick, Journal of the National Cancer Institute, February 2, 2005; Vol. 97: pp. 195–199.

169. 92. N. Leone and D. Courbon, "Zinc, Copper, and Magnesium and Risks for All-cause, Cancer, and Cardiovascular Mortality," Epidemiology 2006; 17 (3): 308–314.

170. C. Skibola, Journal of Nutrition, February 2005; Vol. 135: pp. 296–300. News release, University of California, Berkeley.

171. R. Pokan et al., "Oral Magnesium Therapy, Exercise Heart Rate, Exercise Tolerance, and Myocardial Function in Coronary Artery Disease Patients," British Journal of Sports Medicine 6 July 2006; 40: 773–778; doi: 10.1136/bjsm.2006.027250

172. Teitelbaum, Jacob. From Fatigued to Fantastic: A Clinically Proven Program to Regain Vibrant Health and Overcome Chronic Fatigue and Fibromyalgia New, revised third edition. Penguin Group.

173. 121. D. C. Rushton, I. D. Ramsay, J. J. Gilkes, et al., "Ferritin and Fertility," letter to the editor," The Lancet 337 (8757) (22 June 1991): 1554.

Chapter 12: Fix Your Mitochondria

174. Horowitz, Richard (2017-02-14). How Can I Get Better?: An Action Plan for Treating Resistant Lyme &

Chronic Disease (Kindle Locations 4448-4452). St. Martin's Press. Kindle Edition.

175.   Advanced Nutrition and Human Metabolism (with InfoTrac) by Sareen S. Gropper 4th Edition (April 16, 2004) ISBN: 0534559867: Wadsworth Press. 2. Textbook of Biochemistry with Clinical Correlations by Devlin 6th Edition: ISBN: 0471678082. 3. Food and Nutrients in Disease Management by Ingrid Kohlstadt. CRC Press ISNB: 978-1-4200-6762-0. 4. Resveratrol improves health and survival of mice on a high calorie diet. Baur JA et al. Nature. 2006 Nov 16;444(7117):337-42. Epub 2006 Nov 1.

176.   Therapeutic potential of resveratrol: the in vivo evidence. Baur JA, Sinclair DA. Nat Rev Drug Discov. 2006 Jun;5(6):493-506. Epub 2006 May 26. Review. 6. Diminution of Singlet Oxygen-induced DNA Damage by Curcumin and Related Antioxidants. Subramanian M, et al. Mutat Res. Dec1994;311(2):249-55. 7. Biological activities of Curcuma. Araujo CC, Leon LL.longa L. Mem Inst Oswaldo Cruz. 2001 Jul;96(5):723-8. 8. Effects of oral L-carnitine supplementation on in vivo long-chain fatty acid oxidation in healthy adults. Muller DM, Seim H. Metabolism 2002 Nov;51(11):1389-91. 9. L-Carnitine: therapeutic applications of a conditionally-essential amino acid. Kelly GS. Altern Med Rev. 1998 Oct;3(5):345-60.

177.   Effects of coenzyme Q10 in early Parkinson disease: evidence of slowing of the functional decline. Shults CW, Oakes D, Kieburtz K, et al. Arch Neurol. 2002 Oct;59(10):1541-50.

178.   Fatigue in chronically ill patients. Harris JD. Curr Opin Support PalliatCare. 2008 Sept;2(3):180-6.

179.   Textbook of Natural Medicine (2nd Ed.), Pizzorno JE, Murray MT. Churchill Livingstone, New York, 1999.

180. Complimentary & Alternative Medicines: Professional's Handbook. Fetrow CW, Avila JR. Springhouse, Springhouse, PA, 1999.

181. Botanical Influences on Illness: A sourcebook of clinical research. Werbach MR, Murray, MT. Third Line Press, Tarzana, California, 1994.

182. Incorporating Herbal Medicine Into Clinical Practice. Bascom A. F.A. Davis Co., Philadelphia, 2002.

183. Encyclopedia of Herbal Medicine. Cheallier A. Dorling Kindersley, London, 2000.

184. Pharmacognosy and Pharmacobiotechnology. Robbers JE, Speedie MK, Tyler VE. Williams & Wilkins, Baltimore, 1996.

185. PDR for Nutritional Supplements, 1st Ed. Medical Economics/Thompson Healthcare, 2001.

186. PDR for Herbal Medicines, 1st Ed. Medical Economics/Thompson Healthcare, 1998.

187. The mitochondrial cocktail: rationale for combined nutraceutical therapy in mitochondrial cytopathies. Tarnopolsky MA. Adv Drug Deliv Rev. 2008 Oct-Nov;60(13-14):1561-7. Epub 2008 Jul 4.

188. Beneficial effects of creatine, CoQ10, and lipoic acid in mitochondrial disorders. Rodriguez MC, MacDonald JR, Mahoney DJ, Parise G, Beal MF, Tarnopolsky MA. Muscle Nerve. 2007 Feb;35(2):235-42.

189. R-alpha-Lipoic acid and acetyl-L: -carnitine complementarily promote mitochondrial biogenesis in murine 3T3-L1 adipocytes. Shen W, Liu K, Tian C, Yang L, Li X, Ren J, Packer L, Cotman CW, Liu J. Diabetologia. 2008 Jan;51(1):165-74. Epub 2007 Nov 17.

190. Aging skin is functionally anaerobic: importance of coenzyme Q10 for anti aging skin care. Prahl S, Kueper T, Biernoth T, Wöhrmann Y, Münster A, Fürstenau M,

Schmidt M, Schulze C, Wittern KP, Wenck H, Muhr GM,Blatt T. Biofactors. 2008;32(1-4):245-55.

191.   Antifatigue effect of coenzyme Q10 in mice. Fu X, Ji R, Dam J. J Med Food. 2010 Feb;13(1):211-5.

Chapter 13: Fix Your Constipation

192.   Feldman M., Friedman L.S., Brandt L.J., editors. Sleisenger and Fordtran's Gastrointestinal and Liver Disease. 9th ed., Philadelphia; Saunders: 2010: 259-284

193.   Lembo A., Camilleri M. Chronic constipation. N Engl J Med.. 2003;349: 1360-1368.

194.   Everhart J.E., Go V.L., Johannes R.S., et al. A longitudinal survey of self-reported bowel habits in the United States. Dig Dis Sci.. 1989;34: 1153-1162.

195.   American College of Gastroenterology Chronic Constipation Task Force. Guideline for chronic constipation management. J Fam Pract. 2005;54: 932.

196.   Hsieh C. Treatment of constipation in older adults. Am Fam Physician.. 2005;72: 2277-2284.

197.   Koch A., Voderhoizer W.A., Klauser A.G., et al. Symptoms in chronic constipation. Dis Colon Rectum.. 1997;40: 902-906.

198.   Talley N.J., Jones M., Nuyts G., et al. Risk factors for chronic constipation based on a general practice sample. Am J Gastroenterol.. 2003;98: 1107-1111.

199.   DynaMed: Constipation, Record no. 113862, Ipswich, MA; EBSCO Publishing: 1995.

200.   Rakel, David. Integrative Medicine E-Book (Rakel, Integrative Medicine) (Kindle Locations 37745-37753). Elsevier Health Sciences. Kindle Edition.

Chapter 14: Fix Your Mold

201.   Surviving Mold: Symptoms of Mold Exposure. www.survivingmold.com/mold-symptoms

202.   Ponikau, J.U. et al. "The Diagnosis and Incidence of Allergic Fungal Sinusitis" Mayo Clinic Proceedings 1999 September;74(9):   877-884   DOI: http://dx.doi.org/10.4065/74.9.877

203.   Mycotoxin Detection in Human Samples from Patients Exposed to Environmental Molds Hooper, D.G., Bolton, V.E., Guilford, F.T. and D.C. Straus. Int. J. Mol. Sci. 2009, 10, 1465-1475

204.   Detection of Mycotoxins in Patients with Chronic Fatigue Syndrome Brewer, J.H., Thrasher, J.D., Straus, D.C., Madison, R.A., and D. Hooper. Toxins. 2013, 5, 605-617

205.   Chronic Illness Associated with Mold and Mycotoxins: Is Naso-Sinus Fungal Biofilm the Culprit? Brewer, J.H., Thrasher, J.D., and D. Hooper. Toxins. 2014. Jan; 6(1):66-80

206.   Intranasal Antifungal Therapy in Patients with Chronic Illness Associated with Mold and Mycotoxins: An Observational Analysis Brewer, J.H., Hooper, D., and S. Muralidhar. Global J. of Med. Res. 2015. 15(1). 29-33

207.   Family of Six, their Health and the Death of a 16 Month Old Male from Pulmonary Hemorrhage: Identification of Mycotoxins and Mold in the Home and Lungs, Liver and Brain of Deceased Infant Thrasher, J.D., Hooper, D.H. and J. Taber. Glob. J. of Med. Res. 2014. 14(5). 1-11

208.   A Review of the Mechanism of Injury and Treatment Approaches for Illness Resulting from Exposure to Water-Damaged Buildings, Mold and Mycotoxins Hope, J. The Scientific World Journal. 2013. Article ID 767482. 1-20

209.   Deficient Glutathione in the Pathophysiology of Mycotoxin-Related Illness Guilford, F.T. and J. Hope. Toxins. 2014, 6, 608-623

210.   Detection of Airborne Stachybotrys chartarum Macrocyclic Trichothecene Mycotoxins in the Indoor Environment Brasel, T.L., Martin, J.M., Carriker, C.G.,

Wilson, S.C. and D.C. Straus Appl. Environ. Microbiol. 2005. Nov; 71(11):7376-7388

211. Trichothecenes: From Simple to Complex Mycotoxins McCormick, S.P., Stanley, A.M., Stover, N.A., and N.J. Alexander. Toxins. 2011. 3, 802-814

212. Stachybotrys chartarum, Trichothecene Mycotoxins, and Damp Building-Related Illness. New Insights into a Public Health EnigmaToxicol. Sci. 2008. 104(1):4-26

213. Mycotoxin Production by Indoor Molds Nielsen, K.F. Fungal Genetics and Biology. 2003. 39:103-117

214. Mold and Mycotoxins: Effects on the Neurological and Immune Systems in Humans Campbell, A.W., Thrasher, J.D., Gray, M.R., and A. Vojdani. Advan. In Appl. Microbiol. 2004. 55:375-405

215. Detection of Trichothecene Mycotoxins in Sera from Individuals Exposed to Stachybotrys chartarum in Indoor Environments Brasel, T.L., Campbell, A.W., Demers, R.E., Ferguson, B.S., Fink, J., Vojdani, A., Wilson, S.C., and D.C. Straus Arch. Environ. Health. 2004. Jun; 59(6):317-323

216. Effects of Toxic Exposure to Molds and Mycotoxins in Building-Related Illnesses Rea, W.J., Didriksen, N., Simon, T.R., Pan, Y., Fenyves, E.J., and B. Griffiths Arch. Environ. Health. 2003 Jul; 58(7):399-405

217. Enzyme Immunoassay for the Macrocyclic Tricothecene Roridin A: Production, Properties and use of Rabbit Antibodies Martlbauer, E., Gareis, M. and G. Terplan Appl. Environ. Microbiol. 1988. Jan; 54(1): 225-230

218. Correlation between the Prevalence of Certain Fungi and Sick Building Syndrome Cooley, J.D., Wong, W.C., Jumper, C.A., and D.C. Straus. Occup. Environ. Med. 1998; 55:579-584

Chapter 15: Fix Your Heavy Metals and Chemicals

219. "Breastfeeding as an Exposure Pathway for Perfluorinated Alkylates," Ulla B. Mogensen, Philippe Grandjean, Flemming Nielsen, Pal Weihe, and Esben Budtz-Jørgensen, *Environmental Science & Technology*, August 20, 2015, doi: 10.1021/acs.est.5b02237

220. http://www.ewg.org/news/news-releases/2009/12/02/toxic-chemicals-found-minority-cord-blood

221. Family Wellness HQ (November 2012) "The Most Common Heavy Metals, Their Sources and Their Effects"

222. Doctor's Data. www.doctorsdata.com

223. http://www.my.webmd.com/content/Article/90/10 0860.htm; and E. Oken, R. O. Wright, K. P. Kleinman, et al., "Maternal Fish Consumption, Hair Mercury, and Infant Cognition in a U. S. Cohort," Environ Health Perspect 2005; 113 (10): 1376–1380.

224. Elevated serum pesticide levels and risk for Alzheimer disease. JAMA Neurol. Published online January 27, 2014. doi: 10.1001/ jamaneurol. 2013.6030.

Chapter 16: Fix Your Stealth Infections

225. *Horowitz, Richard. Why Can't I Get Better? Solving the Mystery of Lyme and Chronic Disease. St. Martin's Press. Kindle Edition.*

226. *Borrelia burgdorferi and Treponema pallidum: a comparison of functional genomics, environmental adaptations, and pathogenic mechanisms.* Stephen F. Porcella and Tom G. Schwan Laboratory of Human Bacterial Pathogenesis, Rocky Mountain Laboratories, National Institute of Allergy and Infectious Diseases, NIH, Hamilton, Montana

227. *Antibiotics and increased temperature against Borrelia burgdorferi in vitro.* Reisinger E, Wendelin I, Gasser R, Halwachs G, Wilders-Truschnig M, Krejs G. Department of Medicine, Karl Franzens University, Graz, Austria. Scand J Infect Dis. 1996; 28 (2): 155-7. PMID: 8792482.

228. Columbia University Medical Center: Lyme and Tick-Borne Diseases Research Center: Babesiosis

229. Columbia University Medical Center: Lyme and Tick-Borne Diseases Research Center: Bartonella

230. Columbia University Medical Center: Lyme and Tick-Borne Diseases Research Center: Lyme Disease

231. Forsgren, S. Mycoplasma – Often Overlooked In Chronic Lyme Disease. IMMED Public Health Alert, v. 4, no. 7

232. 3. R. B. Marchesani, "Critical Antiviral Pathway Deficient in Chronic Fatigue Syndrome Patients." Infectious Disease News, August 1993, p. 4.

233. Hook S, Nelson C, Mead P. (2013) Self-reported Lyme disease diagnosis, treatment, and recovery: results from 2009, 2011, & 2012 HealthStyles nationwide surveys. Presented at the 13th International Conference on Lyme Borreliosis and other Tick-Borne Diseases, Boston, MA, August 19, 2013.

234. Identifying Lyme Disease and Other Tick-Borne Illnesses Allen HB, Morales D, Jones K, Joshi S. Alzheimer's disease: a novel hypothesis integrating spirochetes, biofilm, and the immune system. J Neuroinfect Dis. 2016;7: 200. doi: 10.4172/ 2314-7326.1000200.

235. Bu X-L, et al. A study on the association between infectious burden and Alzheimer's disease. Eur J Neurol. 2015 Dec; 22(12): 1519– 25. doi: 10.1111/ ene. 12477.

236. Epub 2014 Jun 9. Clark K, et al. Lyme borreliosis in human patients in Florida and Georgia, USA. Int. J Med Sci. 2013;10(7): 915– 931.

237. Girard YA, Fedorova N, Lane RS. Genetic diversity of Borrelia burgdorferi and detection of B. bissettii-like DNA in serum of north-coastal California residents. J Clin Microbiol. 2011;49: 945– 954.

238. Johnson L, Wilcox S, Mankoff J, Stricker RB. Severity of chronic Lyme disease compared to other chronic

conditions: a quality of life survey. Wilke C, ed. PeerJ. 2014;2: e322. doi: 10.7717/ peerj. 322.

239.   Jung C-R, Lin Y-T, Hwang B-F. Ozone, particulate matter, and newly diagnosed Alzheimer's disease: a population-based cohort study in Taiwan. J Alzheimer's Dis. 2015;44: 573– 584. doi: 10.3233/ JAD-140855.

240.   Miklossy, J. Chronic inflammation and amyloidogenesis in Alzheimer's disease: role of spirochetes. J Alzheimer's Dis. Dec 2004;6(6): 639– 49; discussion 673– 81; J Alzheimer's Dis. (review). May 13, 2008;13(4): 381– 391.

241.   Pritt BS, et al. Identification of a novel pathogenic borrelia species causing Lyme borreliosis with unusually high spirochetemia: a descriptive study. Lancet Infect Dis. 2016 Feb 5. pii: S1473– 3099(15) 00464– 8. doi: 10.1016/ S1473-3099(15) 00464-8. [Epub ahead of print]. Richardson J, et al.

242.   Aguero-Rosenfeld ME, Wang G, Schwartz I, Wormser GP. Diagnosis of Lyme borreliosis. Clin Microbiol Rev. 2005;18: 484– 509.

Chapter 17: Fix Your Sinus Infections

243.   Centers for Disease Control and Prevention National Center for Health Statistics: Vital and health statistics: current estimates from the National Health Interview survey. 1995 Available at http:// www.cdc.gov/ nchs/ nhis.htm

244.   Ponikau J.V., Sherris D.A., Kern E.B., et al. The diagnosis and incidence of allergic fungal sinusitis. Mayo Clin Proc. 1999;74: 877-884.

245.   Rakel, David (2012-04-12). Integrative Medicine E-Book (Rakel, Integrative Medicine) (Kindle Locations 12049-12050). Elsevier Health Sciences. Kindle Edition.

246.   Biotoxin Journey: MARCoNS (updated June 20, 2015)

247.   Rakel, David (2012-04-12). Integrative Medicine E-Book (Rakel, Integrative Medicine) (Kindle Locations 11306-11307). Elsevier Health Sciences. Kindle Edition.

Chapter 19: Fix Your Electromagnetic Frequencies

248.   "Peer-reviewed scientific studies on EMF related subjects" Powerwatch.org

249.   Warren, V. (July 2011) "EMF Exposure: Worse than Cigarettes? The Silent Enemy Harming Your Health Today" Mercola.com

250.   Burrell, L. (April 2015) "Dirty Electricity in the Home Threatens Human Health" NaturalHealth365

251.   Electromagnetichealth.org "Quotes from Experts

252.   The Bio Initiative Report, with 1,800 published studies. bioinitiative.org

253.   Dr. Magda Havas has collected nearly 8,000 published studies on the negative effects of EMF on humans and animals. http://www.magdahavas.com/

254.   Heavy Cell Phone Use Can Quadruple Your Risk of Brain Cancer. (2015). http://articles.mercola.com/sites/articles/archive/2015/01/06/cell-phone-use-brain-cancer-risk.aspx

255.   Samuel Milham (2010). Dirty electricity: electrification and the diseases of civilization. http://amzn.to/2mbr3Mi

256.   Sam Wieder (2015), Unplug: How to Survive and Thrive in a Wi-Fi World Gone Wild. http://amzn.to/2lOAmS0

257.   Dr. Jonathan Halpern (2014) Electromagnetic Radiation Survival Guide: Step by Step Solutions—Protect Yourself & Family Now. http://amzn.to/2lzqHvR

258.   Smart Meters. http://emfsafetynetwork.org/smart-meters/

259.   EMF Meters. http://www.lessemf.com/index.html

260.   StopSmartMeters.org

About the Author

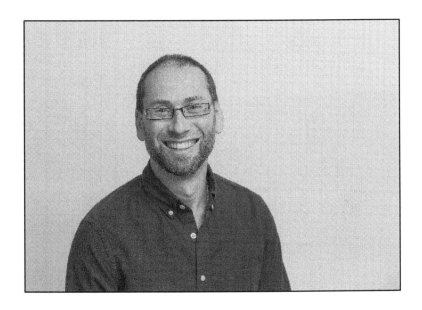

Dr. Evan, as he is affectionately known, is and one of the nation's leaders on finding the root causes of chronic fatigue and resolving them. He suffered from chronic fatigue for five years before he achieved resolution using the Fix Your Fatigue Program that he pioneered at the Hirsch Center for Integrative Medicine in Olympia, Washington. He has helped hundreds of people resolve their chronic fatigue and is on a mission to help 100,000 more through blog articles, online courses, books, 1-on-1 consults and the training of providers. He has lectured nationally and internationally on topics in integrative and functional medicine and is board certified in family medicine and integrative medicine. When he's not at the office, you can find him singing musicals, playing basketball, traveling, dancing hip-hop, and spending time with his wife and daughter.

v2

Made in the USA
Middletown, DE
10 November 2022

14572410R00197